THE HEART-SMART
DIABETES
KITCHEN

Fresh, Fast, and Flavorful Recipes Made with Canola Oil

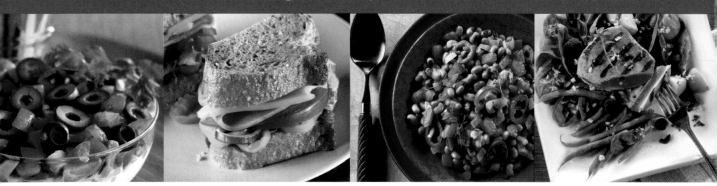

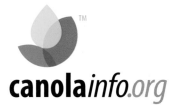

canolainfo.org

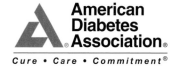

American Diabetes Association
Cure • Care • Commitment

American Diabetes Association

Director, Book Publishing, Robert Anthony; *Managing Editor, Book Publishing*, Abe Ogden; *Project Manager*, Greg Guthrie; *Production Manager*, Melissa Sprott; *Composition and Cover Design*, pixiedesign, llc; *Printer*, R.R. Donnelley.

Canola Council of Canada/CanolaInfo

Vice President, Robert Hunter; *Editor-in-Chief*, Angela Dansby; *Editor*, Kristyn Schiavone; *Assistant Editors*, Maura Comerford, Simone Demers-Collins, Dorothy Long, and Ellen Pruden.

Recipe Development: Nancy S. Hughes

Food Photography: Taran Z Studio
Food Styling: Lisa Cherkasky
Additional Photography: Brian Gould Photography (p. 3, 9, 11, and 15) and Black Box Images (p. 11, bottom image, and 14)

Printed in the United States of America
3 5 7 9 10 8 6 4 2

The suggestions and information contained in this publication are generally consistent with the Clinical Practice Recommendations and other policies of the American Diabetes Association as well as the nutritional guidelines of the Canola Council of Canada, but they do not represent the policy or position of either organization or any of their boards or committees. Reasonable steps have been taken to ensure the accuracy of the information presented. However, the American Diabetes Association and the Canola Council of Canada cannot ensure the safety or efficacy of any product or service described in this publication. Individuals are advised to consult a physician or other appropriate health care professional before undertaking any diet or exercise program or taking any medication referred to in this publication. Professionals must use and apply their own professional judgment, experience, and training and should not rely solely on the information contained in this publication before prescribing any diet, exercise, or medication. The American Diabetes Association and the Canola Council of Canada—including their officers, directors, employees, volunteers, and members—assume no responsibility or liability for personal or other injury, loss, or damage that may result from the suggestions or information in this publication.

♾ The paper in this publication meets the requirements of the ANSI Standard Z39.48-1992 (permanence of paper).

ADA titles may be purchased for business or promotional use or for special sales. To purchase more than 50 copies of this book at a discount, or for custom editions of this book with your logo, contact the American Diabetes Association at the address below, at booksales@diabetes.org, or by calling 703-299-2046.

American Diabetes Association
1701 North Beauregard Street
Alexandria, Virginia 22311

DOI: 10.2337/9781580403313

Library of Congress Cataloging-in-Publication Data
The heart-smart diabetes kitchen : fresh, fast, and flavorful recipes made with canola oil / by American Diabetes Association and CanolaInfo.
    p. cm.
Includes bibliographical references and index.
ISBN 978-1-58040-331-3 (alk. paper)
1. Heart--Diseases--Diet therapy--Recipes. 2. Canola oil. 3. Diabetes--Diet therapy--Recipes.
RC684.D5H445 2009
641.5'6311--dc22
                    2009027208

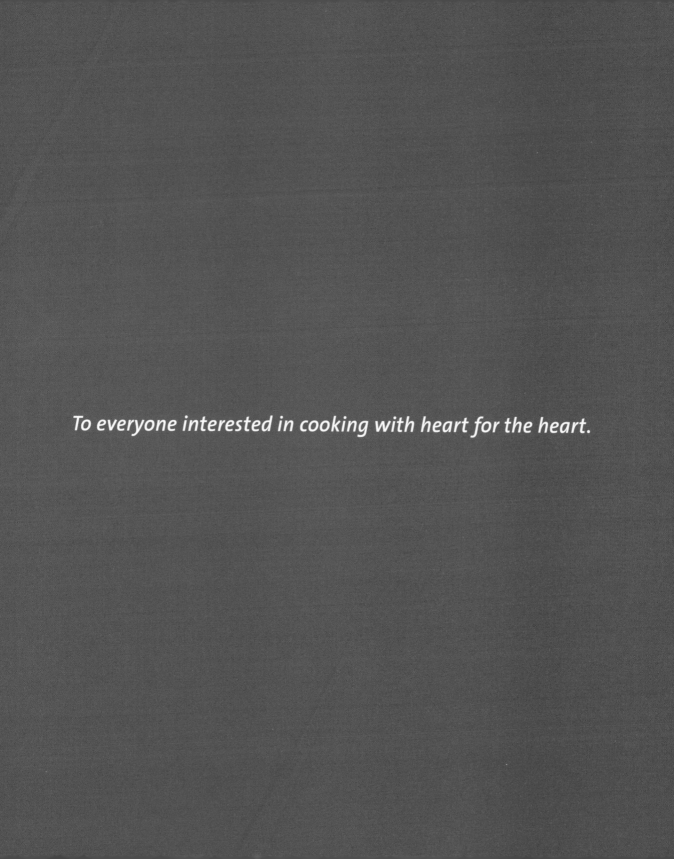

To everyone interested in cooking with heart for the heart.

CONTENTS

INTRODUCTION | **1**

BREAKFAST | **17**

Fresh Herb and Spinach Quiche | 18

Artichoke Frittata with Fresh Vegetable Sauté | 19

Fresh Spinach and Sweet Tomato Omelet with Feta | 20

Sausage and Veggie Breakfast Casserole | 21

English Muffin Pile-Ups | 22

Poached Egg-English Muffin Stacks with Creamy Lemon Sauce | 23

French Toast with Blueberries and Creamy Apricot Sauce | 24

French Toast with Dark Cherry-Pomegranate Sauce | 26

Buttermilk Pancakes with Fresh Strawberry-Orange Topping | 27

Grilled Cinnamon-Pear Sandwiches | 28

Black Bean Tortilla Rounds | 29

Hash Browns with Ham and Chunky Vegetables | 31

Sausage and Country Vegetables on Grits | 32

Banana Bread with Honey Drizzle | 33

Whole-Grain Blueberry Muffins | 34

Oatmeal Breakfast Cookies | 35

Almond Cherry Biscotti with Citrus | 36

Sautéed Apple-Raisin Oatmeal | 38

Creamy Apricot-Mango Smoothies | 39

Canola Granola | 41

LUNCH | **43**

Corn and Skillet-Roasted Poblano Soup | 44

Ham and Lentil Soup with Cloves | 45

Hearty Minestrone with Sausage | 46

Garlic White Bean Soup with Smoked Sausage | 47

Creamy Pumpkin-Apple Bisque | 48

Vegetable Penne Salad with Feta | 50

Bulgur and Rosemary-Edamame Salad | 51

Black Bean, Jalapeño, and Yellow Rice Salad | 52

Grilled Tuna Niçoise Salad | 53

Crunchy Chicken-Cilantro Lettuce Wraps | 55

Spring Greens with Chicken and Sweet
Pomegranate Vinaigrette | 56

Greek Pepperoncini Pitas | 57

Cajun Pile-Ups with Pepper Sauce | 58

Italian-Style Sub with Dijon-Garlic Spread | 60

Turkey-Swiss Panini | 61

Vegetarian Sandwich with Sun-Dried
Tomato Spread | 62

Open-Faced Sloppy Joes | 64

Lentil Tortillas | 65

APPETIZERS | 67

Marinated Italian Vegetable Toss | 68

Spicy Mediterranean White Bean Hummus | 70

Crunchy Red Pepper-Ginger Relish with
Cucumber Rounds | 71

Creamy Black Bean Stack Dip | 73

Mini Potatoes with Caramelized Onions
and Blue Cheese | 74

Soy-Marinated Mushrooms with Cilantro
and Basil | 75

Crispy Baked Zucchini Spears with Lemon | 76

Mini Corn Cakes with Chipotle Aioli | 77

Basil Focaccia Wedges | 79

Mini Vegetable Panini | 80

West Indies Shrimp and Jalapeño Rounds | 81

Pork Sliders with Raspberry Mustard Sauce | 82

Mini Greek Chicken Kabobs | 84

Apricot Hoisin-Glazed Meatballs | 85

SALADS | 87

White Bean and Roasted Red Pepper Salad | 88

Lime-Zested Tomatillo-Black Bean Salad | 89

Sweet Grape Tomato and Poblano Salad | 90

Greek Garbanzo Salsa Salad | 91

Jicama and Sweet Lemon Salad | 93

Fresh Broccoli and Dried Cranberry Salad | 94

Asian Vegetable Slaw | 95

Sweet Pineapple-Ginger Slaw | 96

Baby Spinach and Prosciutto with Sherry
Vinaigrette | 97

Roasted Beet and Carrot Salad | 98

Mixed Greens, String Beans, and Walnuts with
White Wine-Raspberry Vinaigrette | 100

Simple Fresh Herb Salad | 101

Sweet and Crispy Cucumber-Anaheim Salad | 102

Barley-Artichoke Salad on Romaine | 103

Quinoa and Browned Onion Salad with
Apples | 105

Asparagus-Wheat Berry Salad with Blue
Cheese | 106

Wilted Kale Salad | 107

Spinach Salad with Grilled and Fresh Fruit | 108

SIDES | 111

Asparagus with Creamy Dijon Sauce | 112

Black Beans with Green Chile Sauce | 113

Black-Eyed Peas with Jalapeño and Tomatoes | 114

Skillet Broccoli with Tangy Sweet Sauce | 116

Spicy Corn with Poblano Peppers | 117

Stewed Eggplant, Tomatoes, and Fresh Basil | 118

Green Beans with Spicy Mustard Sauce | 119

Turnip Greens with Smoked Sausage | 120

Cumin'd Lentils and Carrots | 121

Garlic Snow Peas with Cilantro | 123

Crispy Crunchy Oven-Fried Okra | 124

Stuffed Portobello Caps with Parmesan Crumb Topping | 125

Baked Acorn Squash with Cranberry-Orange Sauce | 126

Toasted Sesame Seed Quinoa | 128

Yellow Rice and Red Pepper Tosser | 129

Spinach and Mushroom Barley Pilaf | 130

Roasted Root Vegetables with Balsamic Reduction | 132

Sweet Potatoes with Caramelized Sherry Onions | 133

Zucchini Boats | 134

High-Roasted Onions | 135

ENTRÉES | 136

SEAFOOD

Deviled Crab Cakes with Spicy Sauce | **138**

Scallops with Parmesan Pasta | **139**

Grilled Shrimp with Sweet Hot Sauce | **140**

Tuna Kabobs with Mild Wasabi Cream | **141**

Classic Tuna Casserole | **142**

Lime-Infused Halibut with Ginger Relish | **143**

Roasted Salmon with Adobo Cream Sauce | **144**

Sweet Tomato Creole Tilapia | **145**

Fish Tacos with Avocado Salsa | **146**

POULTRY

Baked Chicken Legs with Creamy Honey-Mustard Dip | **148**

Provençal Chicken with White Wine, Garlic, and Apricots | **149**

Grill Pan Chicken with Fiery Mango-Ginger Salsa | **151**

Chicken with Roasted Red Pepper Sauce | **152**

Panko-Parmesan Chicken with Capers | **153**

Sweet Spice-Rubbed Chicken | **154**

Chicken and Artichokes with Pasta | **155**

Jambalaya with Smoked Turkey Sausage and Chicken | **156**

Roasted Turkey with Rosemary and Sage | **158**

Hometown Turkey Meatloaf | **159**

Skillet Turkey Ham with Curried Apples and Onions | **160**

PORK

Thyme-Roasted Pork Loin with Peach-Raspberry Sauce | 161

Pork Tenderloin, Potatoes, and Horseradish-Mustard Seed Sauce | 163

Pork Tenderloin with Sweet Soy Marinade | 164

Pork Medallions with Rich Onion Sauce | 165

Hoisin Orange Pork on Asian Vegetables | 166

Shredded Cajun Pork and Grits | 168

Slow Cooker Smoky Pork Buns | 169

Rosemary Pork Chops with Tomato-Caper Topping | 170

BEEF

Grilled Flank Steak with Balsamic Vinegar and Red Wine | 171

Coffee-Crusted Sirloin Steak | 172

Central American-Style Beef | 173

Beef Tenderloin and Portobellos with Marsala Sauce | 175

Red Wine-Braised Beef with Vegetables | 176

Drunken Beef Goulash | 177

Creamy Beef, Mushrooms, and Noodles | 178

Layered Mexican Casserole | 180

MEATLESS

Barley, White Bean, and Artichoke Toss | 181

Black Bean Burgers with Avocado-Lime Mayonnaise | 183

Black Bean Skillet with Butternut Squash | 184

Sweet Home Chili on Spaghetti Squash | 185

Vegetable Pasta with Tapenade and Pine Nuts | 186

Curried Sweet Potato and Peanut Stew | 188

Toasted Pecan Quinoa with Red Peppers | 190

Sesame Thai Toss with Peanut Lime Sauce | 191

DESSERTS | 193

Glazed Pineapple-Orange Bundt Cake | 194

Mini Fruit Tarts with Cheesecake Filling | 195

Mango-Banana Phyllo Nests | 196

Harvest Pumpkin Pie | 198

Chocolate Mint Pie with Espresso Sauce | 199

Skillet Pie with Oat-Pecan Crumble | 200

Fresh and Dried Fruit Ginger Crumble | 201

Blueberry-Lemon Country Cobbler | 203

Homestyle Shortcakes | 204

Spiced Berry Sauce | 205

Melon Infused with Mint and Lime | 206

Traditional Rolled Sugar Cookies | 207

Toffee-Pecan Topped Cookies | 208

Sticky, Crunchy Cereal Rounds | 210

Apricot-Cranberry Nut Squares | 211

Rich, Warm Brownie Wedges with Java Cream | 212

Chocolate Fondue | 214

INDEX | 215

ACKNOWLEDGMENTS

First and foremost, thank you to our wonderful recipe developer, Nancy S. Hughes, whose impeccable taste, tried-and-true culinary skills, and effervescent personality were a recipe for success with this cookbook. Her zest for life literally carries through to the recipes, which all pop with flavor! Nancy is an established cookbook author, having developed over 4,000 published recipes and written 12 cookbooks, including *The 4-Ingredient Diabetes Cookbook*, *Quick & Easy Low-Carb Cooking*, and *Last Minute Meals for People with Diabetes* for the American Diabetes Association. Nancy is also a huge fan of canola oil, which she says "wakes up the flavors of ingredients."

Another tremendous thanks goes to the CanolaInfo team members, who spent countless hours writing alongside Nancy and editing this cookbook. The American Diabetes Association's book publishing staff also deserves a big round of applause for editing, keeping deadlines cooking, and pulling all of the production elements together.

Also, we are grateful to our visual arts team, including Rikki Campbell Ogden of pixiedesign, whose graphic design gave us this striking layout, and our talented photographer Taran Z and food stylist Lisa Cherkasky, who showcased the beauty of many of Nancy's recipes.

Finally, we are indebted to the North American canola industry, whose financial support underwrote this cookbook and made it possible in the first place. CanolaInfo is supported by North America's canola growers, crop input suppliers, exporters, processors, food manufacturers, and governments.

We are pleased to note that 100% of all sales of this cookbook will go to the American Diabetes Association to further its mission of preventing and curing diabetes and improving the lives of all people affected by diabetes.

In good health and eating,

American Diabetes Association, www.diabetes.org

CanolaInfo, www.canolainfo.org

INTRODUCTION

HAVING A HEART-SMART DIET is one of the most important things you can do for your health. It reduces your risk and improves the management of chronic diseases, such as diabetes, heart disease, stroke, and cancer. Heart disease is one of the leading causes of death around the world. Therefore, it affects us all, at least indirectly. People with diabetes are especially at risk for heart disease and stroke; more than 65% (2 out of 3) of people with diabetes die from these afflictions. Heart attacks also occur earlier in life with diabetes. That's why it's essential for everyone with diabetes to be heart-smart in the kitchen.

With a little planning, meals can be delicious and nutritious as well as easy and economical. Preparing such meals can also be fun for the whole family. It's just a matter of getting healthy ingredients and recipes. Plus, introducing children to nutritious foods at an early age encourages their consumption of these foods as adults.

Many of us consider a healthy diet tough to maintain. We claim that we would eat more nutritious meals if we had the time or money, or better yet, if we got fresh, perfectly portioned meals dropped off at our door or prepared by a personal chef. Of course, how many of us are this lucky? We can't let time and money be excuses for poor nutrition, letting cholesterol or blood glucose spiral out of control, or putting off a weight-loss goal. But we can use what we do have to our advantage through smart grocery shopping and cooking. This cookbook is here to help.

Consider the phrase "fresh, fast, and flavorful." It's the basis of *The Heart-Smart Diabetes Kitchen* and defies the notion that healthy meals are bland and time-consuming. With the recipes inside, your heart and taste buds will be pleasantly surprised.

Why is canola oil in all of the recipes? It has the least saturated fat of all common culinary oils and is free of *trans* fat and cholesterol. As far as fats and oils are concerned, canola oil is the perfect heart-smart choice. It even received a qualified health claim from the U.S. Food and Drug Administration on its potential to reduce the risk of heart disease due to its unsaturated fat content. What's more, canola oil has one of the highest smoke points of all cooking oils at 468°F. This heat tolerance, along with a neutral taste and light texture, makes canola oil extremely versatile. It can be used in just about any culinary application.

These facts make CanolaInfo, *the* source of information for consumers about canola oil, the very proud sponsor of this cookbook. The American Diabetes Association, whose mission is to prevent and cure diabetes and to improve the lives of all people affected by diabetes, was a natural fit as publisher of this cookbook. Together, we hope that you, whether you have diabetes or not, will enjoy our fresh, fast, and flavorful recipes for good health.

HEART-SMART

It's no secret that our fast-paced lives sometimes lead us to fast food and quick fixes for meals. That can turn into a recipe for nutritional disaster if you make it a habit over time. Healthy eating ensures that you get important nutrients, helps control your weight and blood glucose levels, keeps your blood pressure down, and lowers your cholesterol. A heart-smart diet, especially when combined with regular physical activity, can also give you more energy and make you look and feel good inside and out.

TOP 10 RULES FOR HEALTHY LIVING

1. **Variety is the spice (and health) of life.** Enjoy a variety of foods from the following food groups: vegetables, fruits, whole grains, low-fat milk products and alternatives, and lean meat and alternatives. Select the healthiest options available in each group.

2. **Bulk up on produce and whole grains.** Eat mainly vegetables and fruits (5–10 servings per day) and whole-grain, high-fiber products. Good sources of fiber are 100% whole grains, such as oatmeal and brown rice, and fresh produce, especially with peels on. To maximize nutrients, go for the rainbow in produce colors—red, orange, yellow, green, indigo, and violet. In general, the richer the color, the more the nutrients.

3. **Trim away bad fats and eat good ones.** Choose foods and ingredients that are lower in fat, especially saturated and *trans* fats. Trim all visible fat from meat and take the skin off poultry and fish to reduce fat and calories. Instead of deep-frying, try baking, broiling, grilling, roasting, poaching, or sautéing. To get healthy

unsaturated fats in your diet, use canola oil, canola mayonnaise (available in major grocery stores), canola oil cooking spray, and *trans-fat-free* soft margarines.

4. **Go fish.** Eat seafood—preferably fish rich in omega-3 fat, such as salmon, rainbow trout, mackerel, and albacore tuna—two to three times a week.

5. **Plant meat alternatives in your kitchen.** Include meat alternatives, such as beans, lentils, tofu, and tempeh, in your diet more often. Also consider milk alternatives like soy beverages.

6. **Throw salt over your shoulder.** Pass on adding salt to your food to keep blood pressure in check. Instead, season your food with onions, garlic, and fresh or dried herbs and spices (e.g., chiles, parsley, oregano, basil, and cilantro). The American Diabetes Association recommends that adults try to keep their sodium intake at 2,300 mg or less per day and even lower if they have high blood pressure.

7. **Downsize and right-size.** Maintain or achieve healthy weight by being mindful of serving sizes and the number of calories you consume daily. Half of an average 9-inch plate should be filled with colorful veggies, one-quarter with whole grains, and

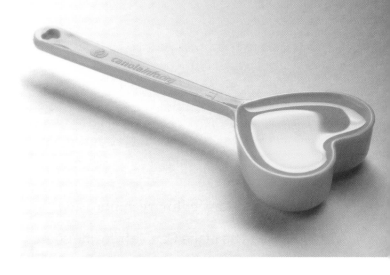

the rest with lean protein. Add a fruit and a glass of milk (or a milk alternative) on the side.

8. **Avoid the grapes of wrath, jitters, and sugar buzz.** Limit your intake of alcohol (one drink for women and two drinks for men daily, if at all), caffeine, sugar, and non-nutritive foods, such as soft drinks and candy.

9. **Be a mover and shaker.** Achieve and maintain a healthy body weight by engaging in regular physical activity. Adults should strive to exercise for 30–60 minutes and children for 60–90 minutes daily.

10. **Smell and dream of the roses.** Minimize stress in your life and get adequate rest. Also, don't smoke. Smoking and exposure to second-hand smoke may increase your risk of developing heart disease and stroke.

FAT FACTS

You need a little fat in your diet for good health. Oils and fats supply energy, carry flavors, and help your body absorb fat-soluble vitamins, like vitamins A, D, E, and K. But make sure it's the right kind of fat—unsaturated. Limit your intake of saturated and *trans* fats, which can negatively impact your cholesterol, thereby increasing your risk of high blood pressure, heart attack, and stroke.

THE GOOD GUYS

Monounsaturated fat

Monounsaturated fat has been shown to improve cholesterol levels. It is found in canola oil, canola mayonnaise, avocados, sesame seeds, olives, and some nuts, such as almonds and hazelnuts.

Polyunsaturated fats

Polyunsaturated fats can lower "bad" LDL cholesterol levels. Two types—omega-3 and omega-6 fats—are considered essential in the diet, because the human body cannot make them on its own. Studies show that omega-3 fat may help protect the heart. The best sources of omega-3s are fatty fish, such as salmon, rainbow trout, and albacore tuna, as well as canola oil, canola mayonnaise, walnuts, eggs enriched with omega-3s, and flaxseed. Omega-6 fat is found in many packaged foods; soybean, sunflower, corn, and cottonseed oils; and sunflower seeds and nuts, such as pecans and Brazil nuts.

THE BAD GUYS

Saturated fat

Saturated fat raises LDL cholesterol. High levels of LDL cholesterol are a risk factor for heart disease. People with diabetes are already at high risk for heart disease, so limiting saturated fat intake can help lower the risk of heart attack and stroke. The American Diabetes Association recommends that no more than 7% of your daily calories come from saturated fat. Foods high in saturated fat include poultry skin, full-fat dairy products, butter, lard, coconut and palm oils, cream sauces, homemade gravy, and fatty meats, such as bacon, hot dogs, sausage, and ribs. Baked products, such as cookies and cakes, can also contain saturated fat.

Trans fat

This artery-clogger raises LDL cholesterol levels and can also lower "good" HDL cholesterol levels for a double whammy. As a result, the American Diabetes Association advises eating as little *trans* fat as possible by avoiding foods that contain it. *Trans* fat is found in stick margarines, some fast foods (e.g., French fries and doughnuts), and some packaged products, such as crackers, cookies, and baked goods. Check nutrition labels for *trans* fat and ingredient lists for partially hydrogenated oils, which are sources of *trans* fat.

Dietary cholesterol

About 20% of the cholesterol in your body comes from the foods you eat. Foods that have high levels of dietary cholesterol include egg yolks, organ meats, shrimp, squid, and fatty meats, so eat them in moderation. Foods high in saturated and *trans* fats also raise your blood cholesterol.

Switching to liquid oils high in monounsaturated fat like canola oil is one of the easiest and most affordable changes you can make to help reduce your risk of heart disease. Use the baking substitution chart on the next page to replace melted solid fat with canola oil in baked goods. This will eliminate *trans* fat and reduce both total and saturated fat without compromising taste.

Comparison of Dietary Fats

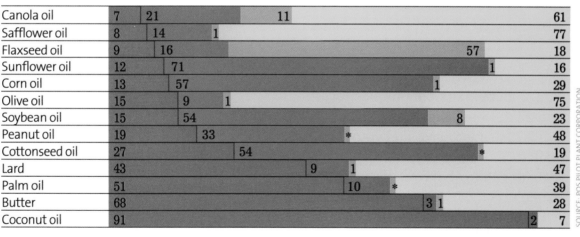

DIETARY FAT

	Saturated fat	Linoleic acid	alpha-linoleic acid	oleic acid
Canola oil	7	21	11	61
Safflower oil	8	14	1	77
Flaxseed oil	9	16	57	18
Sunflower oil	12	71	1	16
Corn oil	13	57	1	29
Olive oil	15	9	1	75
Soybean oil	15	54	8	23
Peanut oil	19	33	*	48
Cottonseed oil	27	54	*	19
Lard	43	9	1	47
Palm oil	51	10	*	39
Butter	68	3	1	28
Coconut oil	91	2		7

SATURATED FAT   POLYUNSATURATED FAT   MONOUNSATURATED FAT

linoleic acid (an omega-6 fatty acid)   alpha-linoleic acid (an omega-3 fatty acid)   oleic acid (an omega-9 fatty acid)

*Trace   Fatty acid content normalized to 100%

SOURCE: POS PILOT PLANT CORPORATION

The colors in this chart show the percentages of fatty acids that make up common oils and solid fats. Red represents "bad" saturated fat and the other colors represent "good" unsaturated fats.

CANOLA OIL BAKING SUBSTITUTIONS	
SOLID FAT (MELTED)	CANOLA OIL
1 cup	¾ cup
¾ cup	⅔ cup
½ cup	⅓ cup
¼ cup	3 tbsp
1 tbsp	2 tsp
1 tsp	¾ tsp

FRESH

Sweet, juicy oranges. Bright red strawberries. Crisp, cool lettuce. Mouthwatering sweet potatoes. You can almost savor these foods by description. Natural foods like these taste so good and are so good for you! Here are some tips for incorporating fresh, healthy ingredients into your meals:

- **Buy produce in season.** Purchasing fruits and vegetables at the "ripe" time is ideal for flavor and your wallet! Not only is seasonal produce loaded with fresh flavor, it is often less expensive at harvest time compared with other times of the year. Buying seasonal produce also adds variety to your menus by forcing you to experiment with the flavors of each season. Learn what grows in your area and when, so you can plan grocery shopping and meals accordingly.

- **Be picky when picking produce.** Odors, bruises, and discolorations are obvious indicators of rotting produce. But price and use-by dates on packaged produce can also help you gauge freshness. Marked-down fruits and vegetables often indicate that they are reaching their peak. Only buy what you can use in a few days.

- **Maximize freshness.** The optimum refrigeration temperature for produce is 40°F, but different types of produce should be stored at different temperatures for the best shelf life, and some should not be refrigerated at all. The coldest part of the fridge should be home to highly perishable items, such as berries, which generally last only 1–3 days. If kiwi, peaches, nectarines, plums, or pears are ripe, they too should be stored with this group (ripening for these fruits is delayed in the refrigerator). Tomatoes, onions, garlic, and most melons are best kept at room temperature in a cool, dark place. Note that apples, peaches, plums, pears, and melons produce significant amounts of ethylene gas, a ripening agent. Unless you want other produce to ripen rapidly, do not keep these items near other fruits and veggies. In addition, onions and potatoes should not be stored together because the moisture in onions can cause potatoes to spoil.

FRESH PRODUCE STORAGE TEMPERATURES	
Apples, berries, broccoli, carrots, cauliflower, celery, grapes, green onions, and leafy greens; and ripe kiwi, peaches, nectarines, plums, and pears.	32–36°F
Bell peppers, yams, potatoes, avocados, cantaloupe, oranges, lemons, and grapefruit.	40–55°F
Tomatoes, onions, garlic, and most melons.	70°F

All cut produce should be stored in the refrigerator.

- **Garden on your windowsill.** Many people don't have the time or space to plant a vegetable garden, but that doesn't mean you have to sacrifice homegrown freshness. A windowsill makes the perfect location for an herb garden. Growing fresh herbs will allow you to conveniently add flavor and freshness to everyday meals like soups and salads, making it easier to turn salt away.

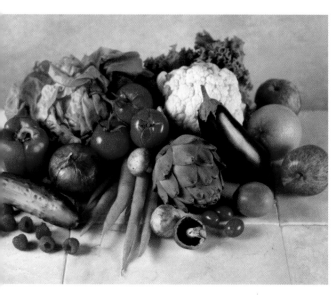

- **Check out local farmers' markets.** If you have the opportunity to buy fresh foods at a farmers' market, take advantage of it! The less travel time from the farm to your plate, the fresher and better the foods taste in general. For example, vine-ripened tomatoes typically have better flavor and texture than artificially ripened tomatoes that are shipped over long distances.

- **Don't let foods expire on you.** Check the expiration dates on perishable products before purchasing them. Note the difference between "sell by" and "use by" dates. "Sell by" means the product is at its peak of freshness by that date. "Use by" literally means "use by this date." Perishable foods without date stamps should be used within a few days or frozen.

- **Select fresh meat wisely.** Raw meat, poultry, and fish should always be your last items to pick up in the grocery store to minimize the time when they're not refrigerated. When selecting them, check out how they are displayed. Fish should be kept on a bed of ice and packaged cuts of any meat should be sealed tightly on refrigerated shelves with no excess moisture on the package and wrap that is entirely clear, not cloudy. If there is red liquid in a package of meat or chicken, it's not a good choice—it means the product has been sitting for a while and is losing its juices. Fresh meat, poultry, and fish should always spring back if you press on the flesh. If you leave a dent, leave it in the store.

- **Store oil properly.** As a key ingredient in the heart-smart kitchen, canola oil should be stored in a cool, dark cupboard for maximum freshness and use. It can last up to a year under these conditions. If in doubt, use your snout and sniff the oil. A rancid or "off" smell means that the oil has oxidized and should be discarded.

- **Make your own dressings and marinades.** Whenever possible, boost your meals with fresh salad dressings and marinades. You can control the flavors, fat content, and quantity with little expense or hassle. There's nothing like a fresh vinaigrette to add pizzazz to greens or vegetables. Canola oil is the perfect base for dressings and marinades due to its neutral taste and light texture. Plus, canola oil is free-flowing at

cold temperatures, so homemade dressings will be ready to serve right out of the fridge. A simple, healthy way to dress 1 cup of greens is with a blend of 1 teaspoon canola oil, 1 teaspoon vinegar or fresh-squeezed lemon juice, and seasonings of your choice.

FAST

Making a heart-smart, home-cooked meal can be easier than it looks. Plus, cooking at home can often be done in less time than eating out and it allows you to better control the ingredients. Try some of the shortcuts below:

- **Make a list.** Grocery shopping without a roadmap often leads to spending money on unnecessary, potentially unhealthy foods. It can also discourage you from preparing those well-intentioned meals, as you may forget some of the ingredients and need to make extra trips to the store. Taking 10 minutes to check out your recipes and pantry and write down what you need can save a lot of time. Plus, if you know what you need, then you can save money by buying ingredients in bulk. With your recipes and ingredients on hand, cooking should be easy.

- **Cook once, eat twice.** Save yourself the trouble of making meals from

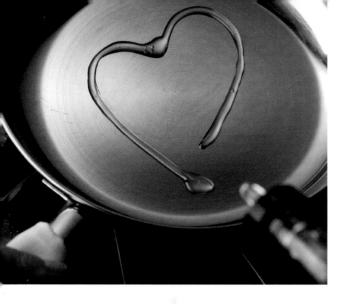

scratch every day and double recipes to allow for two or more servings per person in your family on other days. Most recipes are easy to double and the contents can be safely stored in the refrigerator for 2–4 days or in the freezer. (For best quality, frozen foods should be eaten within 2 months.) And no leftovers are too small to keep—even if there isn't enough for dinner the next night, the leftovers might make a tasty side dish.

■ **Prep your produce.** One of the biggest hassles of using fresh fruits and veggies is that they need to be washed, peeled, seeded, chopped, or all of the above before you start cooking with them. It can be a huge time-saver to wash your produce as soon as you get home and store it in resealable plastic bags. If you already know what you'll be cooking that week, you might even consider

pre-cutting produce accordingly, but be wary of foods like apples and avocados, which oxidize and turn brown if they are cut in advance. Also, don't forget to wash melons and other produce with disposable rinds because bacteria can easily be sliced through from the rinds to the edible flesh.

■ **Thaw without flaw.** If you're using ingredients that need to be thawed, plan ahead and thaw them safely overnight in your refrigerator. You'll be spared a defrosting fiasco right when you're ready to begin cooking. Plus, properly thawing ingredients (particularly meat, fish, and poultry) is a food safety necessity.

■ **"Budget" your time.** In addition to being cheaper than store-bought varieties, homemade sauces, batters, marinades, and dressings are often healthier and require far less fuss than you might expect, especially if you prepare them ahead of time.

■ **Don't get burned out on cooking methods.** When you cook everything the same way, be it sautéing, baking, or grilling, you sacrifice variety in taste and texture. By using multiple preparation techniques for a meal, you'll not only diversify the flavors, but also multitask—a key skill for a speedy chef. For example, place salmon fillets into the oven, make stovetop wild rice, set the table, pour the drinks, and then sauté some spinach in the last 5 minutes of the salmon and rice cooking time. In just 15 minutes, you're ready to eat.

■ **Recycle recipe ingredients.** Remember that a grilled chicken recipe makes a lot more than just grilled chicken. If three of your recipes in a week call for chicken, make a triple batch on the first day you cook and use the ingredient in other dishes. You can use this trick with almost all basic ingredients, from veggies to grains. Just make sure to use refrigerated leftovers within 2–4 days or freeze them instead.

■ **Think fresh, frozen, and canned.** If you can't get fresh produce for a meal or you're in a hurry, use frozen or canned vegetables and fruits as they have similar nutritional value as fresh. Look for products with no added sugar or syrup. If you use canned beans or vegetables, rinse them under water to remove some of the added salt.

■ **Slow cook in the fast lane.** Assemble healthy ingredients in a slow cooker before leaving for the office or going on errands and make a delicious meal that will be ready when you return.

■ **Stock up on healthy ingredients.** Keep your pantry and refrigerator stocked with nutritious staples, so you'll have easy ingredients on hand if you're caught having to improvise. We recommend the following top 10 healthy ingredients for easy cooking:

1. Canned lentils and dry beans (chickpeas, black, kidney)
2. Canned or pouch tuna and salmon
3. Canola oil
4. Eggs
5. Fresh, frozen, and canned fruits and vegetables
6. Lean ground beef
7. Packaged whole grains (e.g., brown rice, whole-grain pasta, and oatmeal)
8. Tofu and tempeh
9. Skinless chicken breasts
10. Tomato or pasta sauce

Finally, don't forget, cooking is like any other skill: the more you do it, the faster and easier it becomes. The recipes in this cookbook, which generally utilize common ingredients and easy cooking techniques, will help fine-tune your cooking skills.

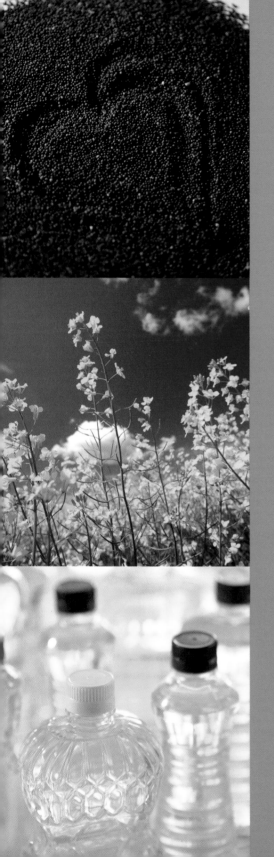

FAST FACTS ABOUT CANOLA

- Canola oil has half the saturated fat of olive oil for a fraction of the price. Canola oil is the best value for health of all culinary oils.

- Canola oil comes from the crushed seeds of canola plants. After harvesting, the seed is sent from a farm to a crushing facility, where the seed is graded and cleaned, and then the oil is extracted, refined, and bottled. Leftover canola solids are processed into meal, which is used as a high-protein livestock feed.

- Canola plants grow from three to five feet tall and produce beautiful small, yellow flowers. The plants produce pods, from which seeds are harvested.

- Canola seeds contain about 42% oil—double the oil content of soybeans. This large percentage of oil comes in a small package; canola seeds are tiny and resemble poppy seeds, though most are brownish-black in color.

- Canola is widely grown in Canada, where it was developed, and to a lesser extent in the United States and Australia. However, canola oil is consumed in many countries.

- Canada—primarily the prairie provinces of Saskatchewan, Alberta, and Manitoba—accounts for the largest supply (exports) of canola in the world.

- Canola belongs to the same family (genus *Brassica*) as broccoli, cauliflower, cabbage, turnip, Brussels sprouts, and mustard. These plants are known as crucifers because they have four-petal flowers resembling the shape of a cross.

- Canola oil is non-allergenic. Food allergens are proteins that can cause the body's immune system to react in susceptible people. Because canola oil does not contain proteins, it will rarely, if ever, cause an allergic reaction.

- Canola oil is a good source of vitamins E and K and plant sterols, which may help protect the heart.

FLAVORFUL

Flavor is the sensory impression of food that you taste and smell, which can stir up emotions. Think of melt-in-your-mouth aromatic steak and mushrooms. Or sweet and savory homemade tomato-basil sauce. And what about the taste of cinnamon- and clove-laced pumpkin pie? The heart-healthy recipes in this cookbook offer unique flavor experiences that will keep your taste buds on their toes without high-sodium, high-fat, or high-calorie foods and cooking methods.

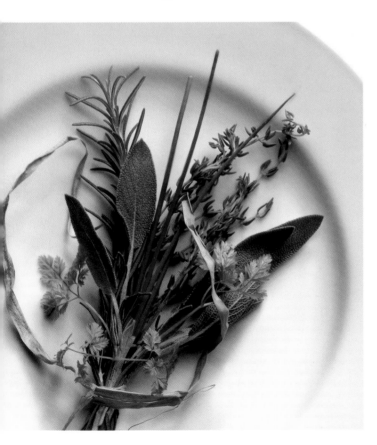

These experiences are created in part through the use of herbs, spices, and bulb vegetables with little to no added salt. Canola oil showcases these seasonings and other ingredient flavors due to its neutral taste and light texture. It enhances, rather than interferes with, food flavors.

THE FAB FOUR OF FRESH HERBS

If you had to pick only four herbs to succeed in the kitchen, we would recommend the following. Of course, these aren't the only herbs with which you'll want to experiment (or that are in our recipes), but keeping some or all of these "fab four" in your fridge or on your windowsill will ensure that culinary dishes pop with flavor every time.

- **Parsley.** Both curly and flat-leaf Italian parsley are very versatile, so they get widespread use in international cuisines. Curly parsley is often used as a garnish, being milder than the flat-leaf type, which is used more for flavoring. Parsley goes with everything—from soups and salads to beef and poultry—but it's famous for its ability to kick up potatoes.

- **Cilantro.** If you're a fan of salsa, chances are you're a fan of cilantro as well. This citrusy herb is primarily found in Mexican, Asian, and Indian cuisines, but it pops up in all sorts of dishes. Cilantro leaves look similar to flat-leaf parsley, so be sure to smell the difference.

- **Oregano.** Pizza lovers know this herb well, as do fans of spicy food. Whereas most herbs used in Italian and Greek cuisine can't stand the heat, oregano's earthy flavor pairs well with acidity and spice. Oregano is frequently combined with tomatoes to balance their flavor or used with basil to create the distinctive flavor of Italian dishes. It's also a staple of Greek food, as it complements olives, lemon, and capers.

- **Basil.** There are many different types of basil, and it is popular in many different types of cuisine. Most common is sweet basil, the star of Italian-inspired dishes. Its fragrant, slightly peppery flavor is typically paired with tomatoes and mozzarella, pizzas, pasta sauces, vegetables, salads, and poultry dishes.

STORING FRESH AND DRIED SEASONINGS

- **Treat fresh herbs like fresh-cut flowers.** It's tempting to return home from the grocery store and toss herbs into the refrigerator as they are. But taking the time to store them properly can give them much longer life. Long-stemmed herbs, particularly those that are grown in warmer climates (such as basil), are best placed in a cup of water and left at room temperature like fresh-cut flowers. Many fresh herbs also fare well when rinsed and wrapped in a paper towel to absorb excess moisture, then stored in a plastic bag or covered loosely with plastic wrap, and refrigerated.

- **Dry or freeze fresh herbs.** Even when herbs are handled properly, they'll still only last about a week. But if you realize early on that you won't be able to use all the herbs you bought, there's still hope. One option is drying them: simply hang the bunch upside down in a cool, dark place for about a week, until the herbs are crisp. Then store the desirable parts in an airtight container. Fresh herbs can also be frozen, retaining their flavor for up to 6 months. Simply remove the leaves from the stems, rinse the leaves, lay them out to dry completely, and store them in the freezer in a resealable plastic bag. Frozen herbs can be added to dishes without thawing, but allow a little extra cooking time or add the herbs sooner in the cooking process.

- **Maximize flavor with dried seasonings.** Dried herbs and spices last much longer if stored in a cool, dark, and dry place, such as a pantry.

Countertop spice racks, while decorative and convenient, are not always the best for storage, depending on the amount of light in your kitchen. And contrary to popular belief, dried seasonings do not last forever. Although they don't spoil, they can lose their flavor strength. Check for expiration dates and remember that whole spices should be used within 4 years and ground spices and leafy herbs within 3 years for peak quality. During these time frames, the ratio of dried herbs to fresh is 1-to-3 in terms of flavor power; in other words, because dried herbs are more concentrated, use one-third the amount called for in a recipe if substituting dried herbs for fresh.

AROUND THE WORLD IN HERBS AND SPICES

Because you probably won't be using a cookbook every time you prepare a meal, it's important to learn different cooking techniques and harmonious ingredient combinations to increase your prowess in the kitchen. You can channel different cultures through your use of seasonings alone! Here are five types of international cuisines that you'll prepare using this cookbook and the seasoning combinations that characterize them.

- **Mexican:** Bell and hot peppers, onion, garlic, lime, cilantro, coriander seeds, cumin, and oregano.

- **Italian:** Basil, bay leaves, garlic, onion, tomato, parsley, oregano, red pepper, and rosemary.

- **Asian:** Soy sauce, hoisin, garlic, ginger, sesame seed, cilantro, lime, orange, and green onion.

- **Caribbean and North African:** Allspice, cloves, coriander seeds, garlic, ginger, curry powder, thyme, oregano, lime, turmeric, cumin, cilantro, and red pepper.

- **Greek:** Olives, dill, garlic, lemon, capers, mint, nutmeg, and oregano.

Prepare for a culinary trip around the world in *The Heart-Smart Diabetes Kitchen*! Enjoy our 151 fresh, fast, and flavorful recipes.

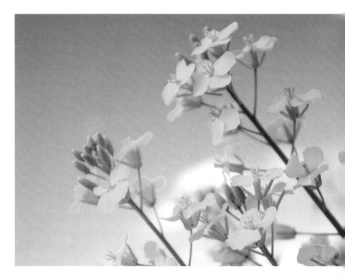

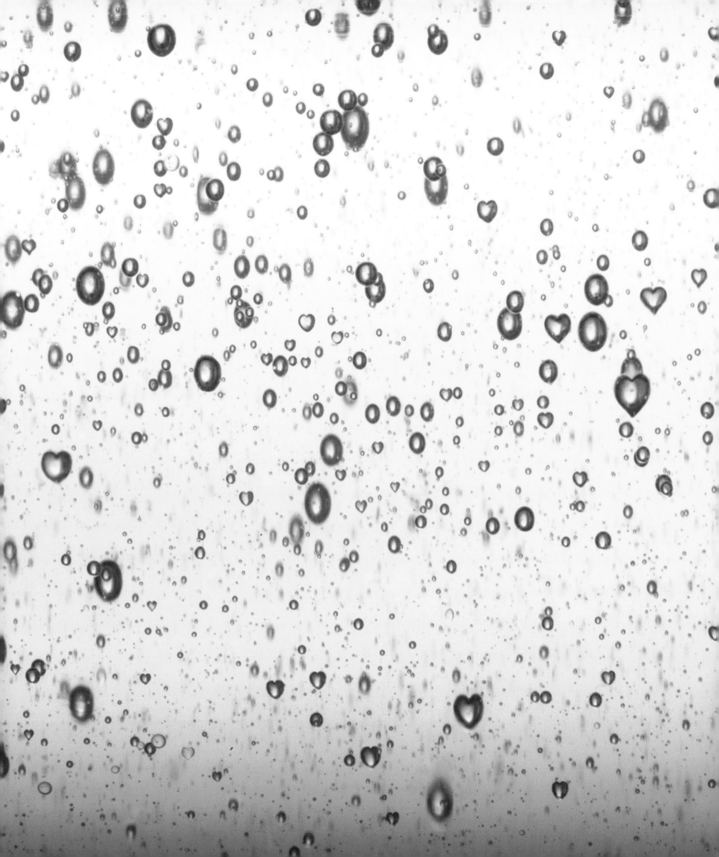

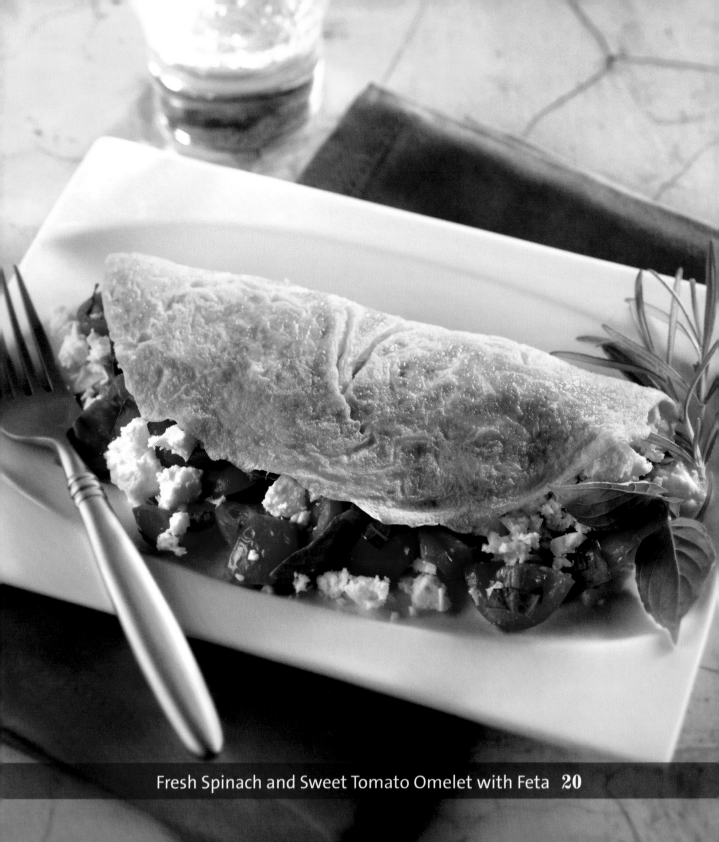

Fresh Spinach and Sweet Tomato Omelet with Feta **20**

BREAKFAST

Fresh Herb and Spinach Quiche | 18

Artichoke Frittata with Fresh Vegetable Sauté | 19

Fresh Spinach and Sweet Tomato Omelet with Feta | 20

Sausage and Veggie Breakfast Casserole | 21

English Muffin Pile-Ups | 22

Poached Egg-English Muffin Stacks with Creamy Lemon Sauce | 23

French Toast with Blueberries and Creamy Apricot Sauce | 24

French Toast with Dark Cherry-Pomegranate Sauce | 26

Buttermilk Pancakes with Fresh Strawberry-Orange Topping | 27

Grilled Cinnamon-Pear Sandwiches | 28

Black Bean Tortilla Rounds | 29

Hash Browns with Ham and Chunky Vegetables | 31

Sausage and Country Vegetables on Grits | 32

Banana Bread with Honey Drizzle | 33

Whole-Grain Blueberry Muffins | 34

Oatmeal Breakfast Cookies | 35

Almond Cherry Biscotti with Citrus | 36

Sautéed Apple-Raisin Oatmeal | 38

Creamy Apricot-Mango Smoothies | 39

Canola Granola | 41

FRESH HERB AND SPINACH QUICHE

YIELD 8 servings | **SERVING SIZE** 1 slice

Fresh basil, rosemary, and spinach make this quiche pop with flavor. It can be made in advance and reheated for meals at any time of day.

CRUST

- ¾ cup all-purpose flour, spooned into measuring cup and leveled
- ¾ teaspoon sugar
- ½ teaspoon salt
- 1 tablespoon fat-free milk
- ¼ cup canola oil

FILLING

- 1 package (¾ ounce) fresh basil leaves, removed from stems
- 1½ teaspoons fresh rosemary leaves, chopped
- ¼ teaspoon coarsely ground black pepper
- ½ cup finely chopped whole green onions
- ½ cup (½ ounce) packed baby spinach
- 2 cups egg substitute
- ½ cup fat-free half and half
- 3 tablespoons capers, drained
- 2 medium plum tomatoes, sliced into thin rounds
- 1 teaspoon canola oil

1 Preheat oven to 425°F.

2 Sift together flour, sugar, and salt. Beat milk into canola oil with a fork until frothy in a small bowl. Form a well in the flour mixture. Add canola oil mixture; combine gently with fork until crumbly. Pat into a 9-inch, deep-dish glass pie pan.

3 Layer ingredients in crust in the following order: basil, rosemary, black pepper, onions, and spinach. Whisk together egg substitute and half and half in a medium bowl and pour evenly over the spinach, completely covering it. Bake 15 minutes.

4 Sprinkle capers over mixture. Arrange tomatoes on top of capers and drizzle remaining 1 teaspoon canola oil evenly over all. Reduce heat to 300°F and bake 35 minutes or until a knife inserted in the center comes out clean. Remove from heat, and let stand 10 minutes before slicing.

Calories 155
Calories from fat 70
Total fat 8.0 g
Saturated fat 0.7 g
Trans fat 0.0 g

Cholesterol 0 mg
Sodium 370 mg
Total carbohydrate 13 g
Dietary fiber 1 g
Sugars 2 g
Protein 8 g

EXCHANGES PER SERVING
½ starch
1 vegetable
1 lean meat
1 fat

Flavorful tip Drizzling a small amount of canola oil over the tomatoes and baking the quiche at a low temperature helps make the tomatoes flavorful and bright in color.

ARTICHOKE FRITTATA
with Fresh Vegetable Sauté

YIELD 4 servings | **SERVING SIZE** ¼ frittata

A frittata is the Italian version of an omelet, which mixes (rather than folds) vegetables and/or meat into eggs. The canola oil in this topping gives a glossy, rich appearance to the vegetables.

2 tablespoons canola oil, divided
1 medium zucchini, thinly sliced
½ cup chopped onion
2 medium cloves garlic, minced
1¼ cups grape tomatoes, halved
1 can (13.75 ounces) quartered artichoke hearts, drained and coarsely chopped
⅛ teaspoon dried red pepper flakes (optional)
¼ cup chopped fresh parsley leaves, divided
1 tablespoon chopped fresh oregano leaves or 1 teaspoon dried oregano leaves, divided
1 cup egg substitute
2 teaspoons red wine vinegar
¼ teaspoon salt

1 Heat 1 tablespoon canola oil in a large nonstick skillet over medium-high heat. Cook zucchini and onion 3 minutes or until lightly browned, using two utensils to toss. Add garlic; cook 15 seconds, stirring constantly. Add tomatoes and cook 2 minutes or until just tender, stirring frequently.

2 Reduce heat to medium, reserve ½ cup vegetable mixture in a separate bowl, and set aside. Stir in artichokes with remaining vegetables in skillet, spread evenly over bottom of skillet, and sprinkle with pepper flakes, half of parsley, and half of oregano. Carefully pour egg substitute over all and immediately reduce to medium-low heat. Cover and cook 10 minutes or until just set. Remove from heat and let stand 10 minutes before slicing.

3 Meanwhile, combine reserved vegetables with vinegar, remaining 1 tablespoon canola oil, remaining parsley, oregano, and salt. Set aside to allow flavors to absorb.

4 To serve, cut frittata into four wedges and top with equal amounts of vegetable mixture.

Flavorful tip The smaller a garlic clove, the more intense the garlic flavor when it is chopped.

Calories 135
  Calories from fat 65
Total fat 7.0 g
  Saturated fat 0.6 g
  Trans fat 0.0 g

Cholesterol 0 mg
Sodium 395 mg
Total carbohydrate 10 g
  Dietary fiber 3 g
  Sugars 4 g
Protein 8 g

EXCHANGES PER SERVING
2 vegetable
1 lean meat
1 fat

FRESH SPINACH AND SWEET TOMATO OMELET
with Feta

YIELD 4 servings | **SERVING SIZE** ½ omelet

Omelets are one of the easiest dishes to prepare and one of the most fun to fill—the possibilities are endless!

- 2 cups egg substitute
- 3 tablespoons fat-free milk
- 2 cups (2 ounces) loosely packed baby spinach
- 2 tablespoons chopped fresh basil leaves
- 1 tablespoon canola oil
- 1 cup grape tomatoes, quartered
- ½ teaspoon chopped fresh rosemary leaves
- Canola oil cooking spray
- ½ cup (2 ounces) reduced-fat feta cheese

1 Combine egg substitute and milk in a medium bowl and whisk until well blended.

2 Place spinach and basil in another medium bowl; set aside.

3 Heat canola oil in a small nonstick skillet over medium-high heat. Add tomatoes and rosemary, and cook 2 minutes or until soft, stirring frequently. Add to bowl with spinach and basil, toss, and cover to allow spinach to wilt slightly and flavors to blend while preparing omelets.

4 Reduce heat to medium. Wipe skillet clean with a damp paper towel. Coat skillet with cooking spray and place over medium heat until hot. Pour half of egg mixture into skillet. Cook 5 minutes; as eggs begin to set, gently lift edge of omelet with a spatula and tilt skillet so uncooked portion flows underneath.

5 When egg mixture is set, spoon half of tomato mixture over half of omelet. Top with half of feta cheese. Loosen omelet with a spatula and fold in half. Slide omelet onto serving plate and cover with foil to keep warm. Repeat with remaining ingredients.

Calories 135
  Calories from fat 55
Total fat 6.0 g
  Saturated fat 1.5 g
  Trans fat 0.0 g

Cholesterol 5 mg
Sodium 445 mg
Total carbohydrate 5 g
  Dietary fiber 1 g
  Sugars 3 g
Protein 16 g

EXCHANGES PER SERVING
1 vegetable
2 lean meat
½ fat

Flavorful tip For variety, place each omelet half in a warmed whole-wheat tortilla and top with 1–2 tablespoons of picante sauce for unique, garden-fresh breakfast burritos!

SAUSAGE AND VEGGIE BREAKFAST CASSEROLE

YIELD 6 servings | **SERVING SIZE** 1 piece (3½-inch square)

This casserole makes entertaining easy, as it must be prepared in advance and the ingredients are simple to assemble.

Canola oil cooking spray

6 slices whole-grain bread, ½-inch thick and torn into ½-inch pieces

4 teaspoons canola oil, divided

½ of 12-ounce package turkey breakfast sausage

1 cup diced green bell pepper

1 cup diced onions

¼ cup water

½ teaspoon dried thyme leaves

½ cup egg substitute

1¼ cups fat-free evaporated milk

⅓ cup (1½ ounces) shredded reduced-fat sharp cheddar cheese

1 Coat an 11 × 7-inch baking dish with cooking spray. Place bread pieces evenly in bottom of dish and set aside. Heat 1 teaspoon canola oil in a large nonstick skillet over medium-high heat, tilt skillet to cover, and cook sausage until no longer pink, stirring frequently. Set aside on a separate plate.

2 Add 1 teaspoon canola oil to drippings in skillet. Cook pepper and onions for 4 minutes or until just beginning to lightly brown on edges. Add water, thyme, and reserved sausage, stirring frequently and breaking up larger sausage pieces, and cook 1 minute or until liquid is almost evaporated. Spoon sausage mixture evenly over bread pieces.

3 Combine egg substitute, milk, and remaining 2 teaspoons canola oil in a medium bowl; whisk until well blended. Pour egg mixture evenly over all. Cover and refrigerate 8 hours or overnight.

4 Preheat oven to 350°F. Remove casserole from refrigerator, uncover, and bake 45–55 minutes or until set and golden. Remove from heat, sprinkle with cheese, and let stand 15 minutes before serving. Do not skip the last step. Standing allows the flavors to absorb and texture to be at its peak.

Fresh tip Adding canola oil to the egg mixture helps distribute moisture evenly throughout the casserole.

Calories 240
 Calories from fat 65
Total fat 7.0 g
 Saturated fat 1.9 g
 Trans fat 0.1 g

Cholesterol 25 mg
Sodium 485 mg
Total carbohydrate 26 g
 Dietary fiber 2 g
 Sugars 9 g
Protein 17 g

EXCHANGES PER SERVING
1 starch
½ fat-free milk
1 vegetable
1 lean meat
1 fat

ENGLISH MUFFIN PILE-UPS

YIELD 4 servings | **SERVING SIZE** 1 muffin half

Wake up to big flavors in every bite of these breakfast stacks.

- 2 whole-wheat English muffins, halved
- ½ cup finely chopped roasted peppers
- 2 teaspoons coarse-grain Dijon mustard
- ⅛ teaspoon dried red pepper flakes
- 3 teaspoons canola oil, divided
- 1 cup egg substitute
- 2 tablespoons chopped fresh basil leaves
- ¼ cup (1 ounce) grated Parmesan cheese

1 Toast muffins in toaster. Meanwhile, combine roasted peppers, mustard, and pepper flakes with 2 teaspoons canola oil in a small bowl.

2 Heat remaining 1 teaspoon canola oil in a medium nonstick skillet over medium heat and tilt skillet to lightly coat bottom. Add egg substitute and sprinkle with basil. Cook, stirring occasionally, until done, about 2 minutes.

3 To assemble, place muffin halves on serving platter and top with equal amounts of red pepper mixture, followed by egg mixture, and sprinkle with cheese.

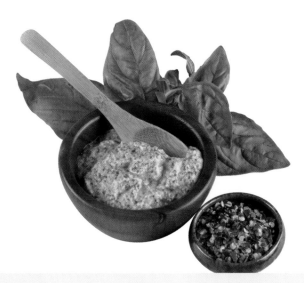

Calories 160
 Calories from fat 55
Total fat 6.0 g
 Saturated fat 1.4 g
 Trans fat 0.0 g

Cholesterol 5 mg
Sodium 415 mg
Total carbohydrate 16 g
 Dietary fiber 3 g
 Sugars 5 g
Protein 12 g

EXCHANGES PER SERVING
1 starch
1 lean meat
1 fat

POACHED EGG-ENGLISH MUFFIN STACKS
with Creamy Lemon Sauce

YIELD 4 servings | **SERVING SIZE** 1 muffin stack

Instead of eggs benedict, this recipe could be called "eggs benefit," as it is a healthier version of the classic dish. A canola mayonnaise sauce replaces hollandaise, which is traditionally made with butter and egg yolks.

SAUCE

2 tablespoons canola mayonnaise

1 teaspoon lemon zest

3 tablespoons plain nonfat yogurt or fat-free sour cream

1 tablespoon fat-free milk

MUFFIN STACKS

Canola oil cooking spray

2 whole-wheat English muffins, split in half (4 rounds)

4 slices Canadian bacon

1 large tomato, cut into 4 slices

3 cups water

4 large eggs

4 teaspoons coarse-grain Dijon mustard

Coarsely ground black pepper (optional)

1 Preheat broiler. Whisk together sauce ingredients in a small saucepan and set aside. Place muffins, bacon slices, and tomato slices in single layer (side by side) on a foil-lined baking sheet coated with cooking spray; set aside.

2 Coat a medium nonstick skillet with cooking spray, add water, and bring to a boil over medium-high heat. Reduce heat to simmering and break one egg in a measuring cup. Carefully slide egg into simmering water, holding the lip of the measuring cup as close to the water as possible. Repeat with remaining eggs, allowing each egg equal space. Simmer eggs, uncovered, 3–5 minutes or until whites are completely set and yolks begin to thicken but are not hard. Baste eggs with water to create a light film over top. Coat a dinner plate with cooking spray, remove eggs with a slotted spoon, and place on plate.

3 Meanwhile, place baking sheet with muffins, bacon, and tomatoes under the broiler 2–3 minutes or until muffins are lightly toasted. Place saucepan with sauce mixture over medium-low heat to warm slightly, but do not bring to a boil.

4 Remove baking sheet from broiler, spoon 1 teaspoon mustard on each muffin half, and place on four dinner plates. Top with warmed bacon and tomatoes. Slide egg on top of each stack and spoon 1 tablespoon sauce over each. Sprinkle with coarsely ground black pepper.

Fast tip Coating a dinner plate with canola oil cooking spray helps the eggs slide off the plate easily.

Calories 225	Cholesterol 225 mg
Calories from fat 90	Sodium 765 mg
Total fat 10.0 g	Total carbohydrate 18 g
Saturated fat 2.3 g	Dietary fiber 3 g
Trans fat 0.0 g	Sugars 6 g
	Protein 16 g

EXCHANGES PER SERVING

1 starch

2 medium-fat meat

FRENCH TOAST
with Blueberries and Creamy Apricot Sauce

YIELD 4 servings | **SERVING SIZE** 2 slices

The secret ingredient in this citrusy French toast is the orange zest. Also, the blueberries contrast beautifully with the peach hues of the toast and sauce.

Canola oil cooking spray

TOAST

2 tablespoons canola oil, divided

1¼ cups egg substitute

¼ cup fat-free milk

1 teaspoon orange zest

1 teaspoon vanilla extract

½ of 16-ounce loaf whole-grain Italian bread, cut diagonally into 8 slices, divided

SAUCE

1 container (6 ounces) fat-free or low-fat vanilla yogurt

3 tablespoons apricot fruit spread

1 teaspoon orange zest

1 cup fresh (or thawed frozen) blueberries

1 Place a large nonstick skillet over medium heat until hot. Coat skillet with cooking spray, add 1 tablespoon canola oil, and tilt skillet to lightly coat bottom.

2 Pour egg substitute, milk, zest, and vanilla into a 13 × 9-inch baking pan. Add four bread slices and turn several times to coat evenly. Place these bread slices in the skillet; cook 3 minutes on each side or until golden. Set aside on a separate plate and cover to keep warm. Repeat with remaining bread slices and canola oil.

3 Combine yogurt, fruit spread, and zest in a blender. Secure with lid and purée until well blended.

4 To serve, place two slices of French toast on each of four dinner plates, spoon equal amounts of yogurt mixture on each slice, and top with blueberries.

		EXCHANGES PER SERVING	
Calories 330	Cholesterol 0 mg		
Calories from fat 80	Sodium 505 mg	2 starch	*Flavorful tip* Working in two
Total fat 9.0 g	Total carbohydrate 46 g	1 fruit	batches keeps the bread from
Saturated fat 1.0 g	Dietary fiber 3 g	1 lean meat	getting crowded, so it can brown
Trans fat 0.0 g	Sugars 15 g	1 fat	properly and create a slight crust.
	Protein 15 g		

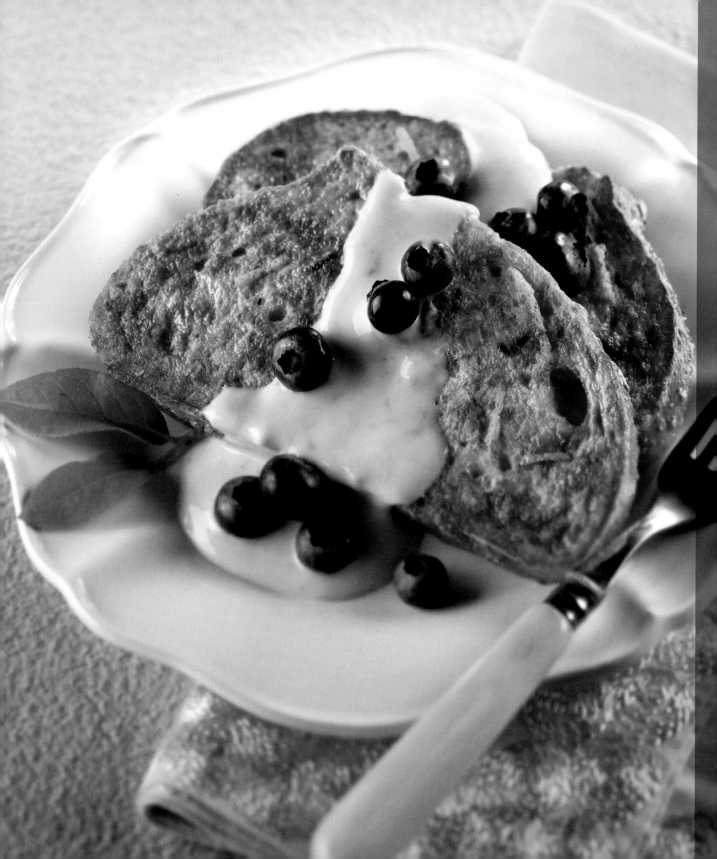

FRENCH TOAST
with Dark Cherry-Pomegranate Sauce

YIELD 4 servings | **SERVING SIZE** 2 slices

Whether you're entertaining overnight guests or starting a special day, this is definitely a recipe to enjoy. Plus, you'll get a dose of antioxidants from the fruit!

Canola oil cooking spray

TOAST
1 large egg
2 egg whites
1/2 cup fat-free milk
1 tablespoon canola oil
1 teaspoon vanilla extract
1/2 of 16-ounce loaf whole-grain Italian bread, cut diagonally into 8 slices
2 teaspoons ground cinnamon

SAUCE
1 cup pomegranate juice
2 teaspoons cornstarch
1 1/2 cups frozen dark sweet cherries
2–3 tablespoons sugar substitute
1/2 teaspoon vanilla extract
1/2 cup fat-free sour cream

1 Preheat oven to 450°F. Coat nonstick baking sheet with cooking spray and set aside.

2 Combine egg, egg whites, milk, canola oil, and vanilla in a small bowl and whisk until well blended. Place bread in a 13 × 9-inch baking pan, pour egg mixture over all, and turn several times until bread slices are completely coated and all egg mixture is used. Place bread slices on the baking sheet, sprinkle evenly with 1 teaspoon cinnamon, and bake 8 minutes; then turn, sprinkle with remaining cinnamon, and bake 7 minutes or until golden.

3 Meanwhile, combine juice with cornstarch in a medium saucepan, whisk until cornstarch is dissolved, and stir in cherries. Bring to a boil over medium-high heat and boil for 1 full minute. Remove from heat. Add sugar substitute and vanilla. Cover to keep warm.

4 To serve, top each serving of French toast with equal amounts of cherry sauce and sour cream.

		EXCHANGES PER SERVING
Calories 375	Cholesterol 55 mg	2 starch
Calories from fat 65	Sodium 355 mg	2 fruit
Total fat 7.0 g	Total carbohydrate 64 g	1 lean meat
Saturated fat 1.1 g	Dietary fiber 6 g	1 fat
Trans fat 0.0 g	Sugars 28 g	
	Protein 13 g	

Fast tip Using a 13 × 9-inch baking pan makes it easier to coat the bread slices evenly.

BUTTERMILK PANCAKES
with Fresh Strawberry-Orange Topping

YIELD 4 servings | **SERVING SIZE** 2 pancakes + ⅓ cup topping

Combining all-purpose flour with white whole-wheat flour gives these pancakes a lighter texture while boosting their dietary fiber. The fresh strawberries and orange zest infuse them with flavor.

PANCAKES
- ½ cup all-purpose flour, spooned into measuring cup and leveled
- ½ cup white whole-wheat flour, spooned into measuring cup and leveled
- 1 tablespoon sugar
- 1 teaspoon baking powder
- ¼ teaspoon baking soda
- ¼ teaspoon salt
- 1 cup low-fat buttermilk
- 1½ tablespoons canola oil
- 2 egg whites

TOPPING
- 2 cups quartered strawberries
- 2 tablespoons water
- 1½ tablespoons sugar
- 1 tablespoon canola oil
- 1½ teaspoons vanilla
- ½ teaspoon orange zest
- ½ cup fat-free sour cream or plain nonfat yogurt

Canola oil cooking spray

1 Combine flours, sugar, baking powder, baking soda, and salt in a large bowl with a whisk. Then whisk together buttermilk, canola oil, and egg whites in a small bowl. Add to flour mixture, stirring until just moist. Let stand 15 minutes.

2 Meanwhile, preheat oven to 200°F. Combine topping ingredients, except the sour cream, in a medium bowl and mash slightly with a fork until a thick consistency is achieved.

3 Heat a large nonstick skillet coated with cooking spray over medium heat. Working in two batches, spoon about ¼ cup batter per pancake onto skillet. Cook 2 minutes or until tops are covered with bubbles and edges look cooked. Turn and cook 2 minutes longer or until pancakes are slightly puffed and golden. Place on a serving platter in the oven to keep warm while cooking remaining pancakes

4 To serve, spoon equal amounts of topping on pancakes and dollop with sour cream.

Fast tip Cartons of egg whites are in the dairy section of grocery stores or you can separate your own. Crack an egg and toss the yolk back and forth between the shells over a bowl. Let the egg white fall into the mixture and discard the yolk and shells.

Calories 305	Cholesterol 5 mg	**EXCHANGES PER SERVING**
Calories from fat 90	Sodium 425 mg	1½ starch
Total fat 10.0 g	Total carbohydrate 42 g	1 fruit
Saturated fat 1.1 g	Dietary fiber 4 g	½ fat-free milk
Trans fat 0.0 g	Sugars 17 g	1½ fat
	Protein 10 g	

GRILLED CINNAMON-PEAR SANDWICHES

YIELD 4 servings | **SERVING SIZE** 1 sandwich

These sweet, unusual sandwiches are a fun way to start the day. They also make a great mid-day snack.

- ¼ cup (2 ounces) fat-free cream cheese, soft tub variety
- 8 slices whole-grain raisin bread
- 1 tablespoon apricot fruit spread
- 1 teaspoon fresh grated ginger
- 1 medium firm green pear, halved, cored, and sliced (6 ounces)
- 1 tablespoon canola oil

1 Spread cream cheese on four bread slices. Place fruit spread in a small microwave-safe bowl. Microwave on high 15–20 seconds or until slightly melted. Stir in ginger. Place 1 teaspoon spread on each bread slice, spreading evenly over all with the back of a spoon.

2 Arrange pear slices on top, overlapping slightly, and top with remaining bread slices.

3 Heat canola oil in a large nonstick skillet over medium heat. Tilt skillet to lightly coat bottom. Add sandwiches; cook 2–3 minutes on each side or until bread is golden. Serve warm.

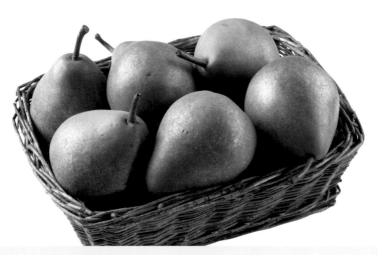

Calories 220	Cholesterol 0 mg	**EXCHANGES PER SERVING**
Calories from fat 55	Sodium 285 mg	
Total fat 6.0 g	Total carbohydrate 38 g	2 starch
Saturated fat 0.8 g	Dietary fiber 4 g	½ fruit
Trans fat 0.0 g	Sugars 18 g	1 fat
	Protein 7 g	

BLACK BEAN TORTILLA ROUNDS

This creamy bean mixture is full of fresh lime and cilantro flavors.

- 4 white corn tortillas
- 1 can (15 ounces) black beans, rinsed and drained
- 1/3 cup medium picante sauce, divided
- 3 teaspoons canola oil, divided
- 2 tablespoons water
- 2 tablespoons fresh lime juice
- 1 teaspoon ground cumin
- 1 cup egg substitute
- 1/4 cup chopped fresh cilantro leaves
- 1/2 cup fat-free sour cream
- 1 medium lime, quartered

1 Preheat oven to 350°F. Place tortillas on a large baking sheet; set aside.

2 Place beans, 1/4 cup picante sauce, 2 teaspoons canola oil, water, lime juice, and cumin in a blender. Secure lid tightly and purée until smooth. Spoon equal amounts of puréed mixture on each tortilla and spread mixture as close to the edge of the tortillas as possible. Bake 8 minutes or until heated through.

3 Meanwhile, heat remaining 1 teaspoon canola oil in a medium nonstick skillet. Tilt skillet to lightly coat bottom, add egg substitute, and cook 2–3 minutes or until done, lightly lifting edges to allow runny eggs to cook.

4 To serve, place tortilla on each of four dinner plates and top with equal amounts of cooked egg, cilantro, sour cream, and remaining picante sauce. Serve with lime wedges.

Fast tip In a rush? Save a step and omit the egg substitute from this dish completely.

Calories 230	Cholesterol 5 mg	**EXCHANGES PER SERVING**
Calories from fat 40	Sodium 390 mg	
Total fat 4.5 g	Total carbohydrate 30 g	2 starch
Saturated fat 0.5 g	Dietary fiber 7 g	1 lean meat
Trans fat 0.0 g	Sugars 4 g	1/2 fat
	Protein 15 g	

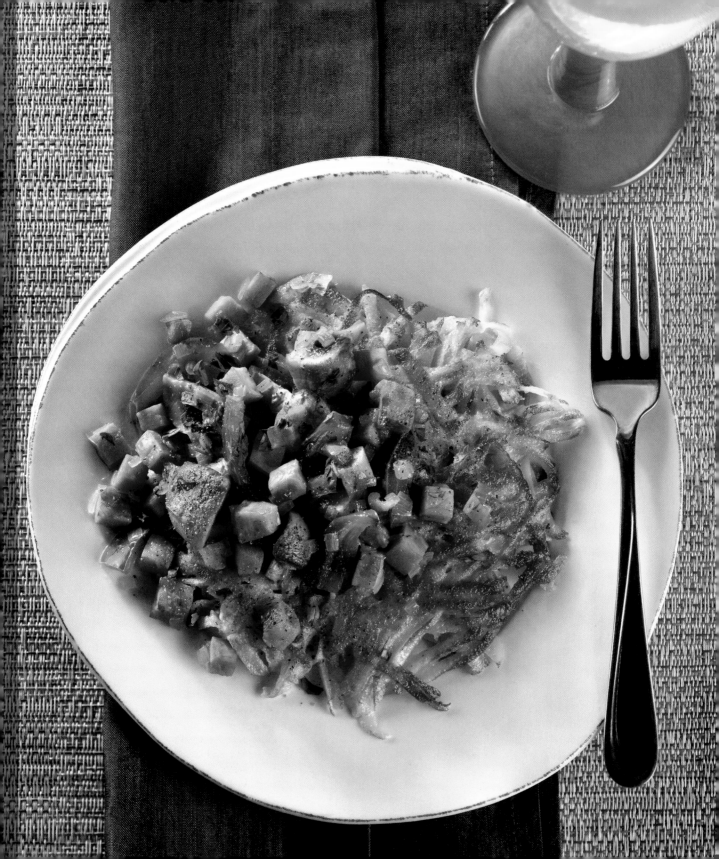

HASH BROWNS
with Ham and Chunky Vegetables

YIELD 4 servings | **SERVING SIZE** 1 hash brown

This hot and hearty fare will bring comfort with every bite.

HASH BROWNS

- 2 medium baking potatoes (12 ounces total), shredded, rinsed, and patted dry with paper towels
- ¼ cup finely chopped onion
- 2 large egg whites
- ⅛ teaspoon salt
- 2 tablespoons canola oil

TOPPING

- Canola oil cooking spray
- 1¼ cups (6 ounces) diced lean ham
- ½ of 8-ounce package whole mushrooms, quartered
- 1 large shallot, finely chopped
- ½ of medium green bell pepper, thinly sliced, and cut into 2-inch-long pieces
- ¼ cup chopped fresh parsley leaves
- Pepper, to taste

1 Combine potatoes with onions, egg whites, and salt in a medium bowl.

2 Heat canola oil in a large skillet over medium-high heat until hot and spoon potato mixture into four mounds in the skillet. Press down lightly on mounds with back of a spatula to level, making patties about 4 inches in diameter. Cook, uncovered, 7 minutes or until bottom is crisp. Gently turn and cook 6–7 minutes or until golden.

3 Meanwhile, place a medium skillet over medium-high heat until hot and coat with cooking spray. Add ham, cook, and set aside. Re-coat same skillet with cooking spray and add mushrooms, shallot, and bell pepper. Coat vegetables with cooking spray and cook 3 minutes or until they just begin to richly brown on edges. Add ham, cover, and set aside.

4 When potatoes are cooked, place on individual plates and spoon equal amounts of mushroom mixture on top of each. Sprinkle with parsley and pepper.

Fresh tip Shred the potatoes first, then rinse and pat them dry before adding the other ingredients, allowing the egg white mixture to adhere to the potatoes. Lightly coating the other vegetables with canola oil cooking spray keeps them moist and browns them evenly.

Calories 225	Cholesterol 20 mg	**EXCHANGES PER SERVING**
Calories from fat 70	Sodium 565 mg	1½ starch
Total fat 8.0 g	Total carbohydrate 25 g	1 vegetable
Saturated fat 0.8 g	Dietary fiber 3 g	1 lean meat
Trans fat 0.0 g	Sugars 3 g	1 fat
	Protein 13 g	

SAUSAGE AND COUNTRY VEGETABLES ON GRITS

YIELD 4 servings | **SERVING SIZE** ½ cup grits + ½ cup sausage mixture

A Southern comfort food, grits are a great base for your favorite breakfast meats and veggies. Grits are also delicious served alone with a little hot sauce.

½ cup quick-cooking yellow grits

3 teaspoons canola oil, divided

¼ lb smoked turkey sausage, thinly sliced

½ cup thinly sliced red bell pepper

½ cup chopped onion

1 medium yellow squash, diced

¼ cup water

2 teaspoons hot pepper sauce

1 Cook grits according to package directions, omitting any salt or fat.

2 Meanwhile, heat 1 teaspoon canola oil in a large nonstick skillet over medium-high heat until hot. Tilt skillet to lightly coat bottom, add sausage, and cook until browned, stirring frequently. Set aside on a separate plate.

3 Add remaining 2 teaspoons canola oil to skillet and cook pepper, onion, and squash 4 minutes or until vegetables begin to lightly brown, stirring frequently. Add water, pepper sauce, and sausage; cook 30 seconds to thicken slightly. Serve sausage mixture over grits with additional hot pepper sauce on side.

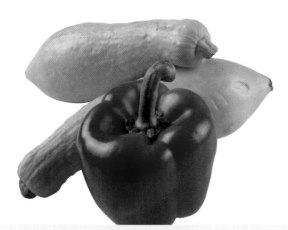

Calories 165
  Calories from fat 55
Total fat 6.0 g
  Saturated fat 1.3 g
  Trans fat 0.0 g

Cholesterol 20 mg
Sodium 275 mg
Total carbohydrate 20 g
  Dietary fiber 2 g
  Sugars 3 g
Protein 7 g

EXCHANGES PER SERVING
1 starch
1 vegetable
1 fat

Fast tip Only a small amount of canola oil is needed to brown the sausage. Because there may be water in the sausage itself, too much canola oil may cause it to splatter.

BANANA BREAD WITH HONEY DRIZZLE

YIELD 12 servings | **SERVING SIZE** 1 slice, about ¾-inch thick

Enjoy a slice of warm bread with a glass of cold fat-free milk for a quick and satisfying breakfast.

1½ cups all-purpose flour, spooned into measuring cups and leveled

1 cup quick-cooking oats

1 teaspoon ground cinnamon

¾ teaspoon baking soda

½ teaspoon salt

¼ teaspoon ground nutmeg

3 very ripe medium bananas, mashed (1½ cups total)

⅓ cup low-fat buttermilk

4 egg whites or ½ cup egg substitute

⅓ cup brown sugar substitute blend

3 tablespoons canola oil

2 teaspoons vanilla extract

Canola oil cooking spray

¼ cup (1 ounce) chopped pecans

1 tablespoon honey

1 Preheat oven to 350°F. Combine flour, oats, cinnamon, baking soda, salt, and nutmeg in a medium bowl.

2 Combine bananas, buttermilk, eggs, brown sugar blend, canola oil, and vanilla in another medium bowl. Stir until well blended. Add to flour mixture and stir until just blended. Do not overmix. Batter will be very thick.

3 Coat a 9 × 5-inch nonstick loaf pan with cooking spray. Add batter and top with pecans. Bake 50 minutes or until a wooden pick inserted in the center comes out clean. Let stand 10 minutes before removing from pan; place on a wire rack to cool completely for peak flavors. Place on a serving tray and drizzle with honey.

Flavorful tip As with most quick breads, this bread is even better the next day because it has had time to meld the flavors.

Calories 195
Calories from fat 55
Total fat 6.0 g
Saturated fat 0.6 g
Trans fat 0.0 g

Cholesterol 0 mg
Sodium 205 mg
Total carbohydrate 31 g
Dietary fiber 2 g
Sugars 11 g
Protein 4 g

EXCHANGES PER SERVING
2 carbohydrate
1 fat

WHOLE-GRAIN BLUEBERRY MUFFINS

YIELD 12 servings | **SERVING SIZE** 1 muffin

These muffins have whole-wheat flour, wheat bran, and oats all in one! They are a more filling and nutritious twist on the classic recipe.

Canola oil cooking spray

1 cup plus 1 tablespoon white whole-wheat flour, spooned into measuring cup and leveled, divided

¼ cup wheat bran

½ teaspoon baking soda

1 teaspoon ground cinnamon

½ teaspoon ground allspice (optional)

½ teaspoon salt

1½ cups quick-cooking oats

1 cup low-fat buttermilk

½ cup sugar

¼ cup canola oil

¼ cup egg substitute

1 tablespoon orange zest

1 cup fresh (or thawed frozen) blueberries

1 Preheat oven to 350°F. Spray a 12-cup nonstick muffin pan with cooking spray.

2 Whisk together 1 cup flour, bran, baking soda, cinnamon, allspice, and salt in a large bowl. Stir in oats.

3 Whisk together buttermilk, sugar, canola oil, egg substitute, and zest in a medium bowl. Stir buttermilk mixture into flour mixture until just blended. Do not overmix.

4 Toss blueberries with remaining flour and fold into batter. Spoon into muffin cups, filling each cup about ⅔ full. Bake 18 minutes. Cool in pan 5 minutes. Remove from pan; serve warm or let cool to room temperature.

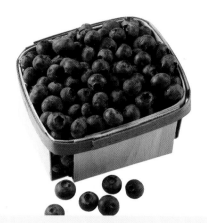

Calories 175
Calories from fat 55
Total fat 6.0 g
  Saturated fat 0.6 g
  Trans fat 0.0 g

Cholesterol 0 mg
Sodium 180 mg
Total carbohydrate 28 g
  Dietary fiber 3 g
  Sugars 11 g
  Protein 4 g

EXCHANGES PER SERVING
2 carbohydrate
1 fat

Fast tip These muffins make a great "brown-bag" snack and taste just as delicious the next day. They also freeze well.

OATMEAL BREAKFAST COOKIES

YIELD 8 servings | **SERVING SIZE** 2 cookies

These cookies are the breakfast of champions! Each serving offers 2 grams of fiber.

1½ cups quick-cooking oatmeal

⅔ cup all-purpose flour, spooned into measuring cup and leveled

⅓ cup wheat bran

2 teaspoons ground cinnamon

½ teaspoon baking powder

¼ teaspoon salt

⅓ cup canola oil

¼ cup egg substitute

1 teaspoon vanilla extract

¼ cup brown sugar substitute blend

½ of large Granny Smith apple, cored and finely chopped (¾ cup)

⅓ cup raisins

Canola oil cooking spray

1 Preheat oven to 375°F. Combine oatmeal, flour, bran, cinnamon, baking powder, and salt in a large bowl. Stir until well blended and set aside.

2 Combine canola oil, egg substitute, vanilla, and brown sugar in a medium bowl. Whisk until well blended and fold in apples and raisins. Add wet mixture to dry mixture and stir until well blended.

3 Using half of the cookie dough, spoon 12 mounds (about 2 tablespoons each) about 1–2 inches apart onto a cookie sheet coated with cooking spray (you may need to lightly shape with your fingertips). Bake 7 minutes or until almost set and slightly firm to touch. Do not cook longer. Note that cookies will not appear done at this point, but they will continue to cook while cooling. Remove from oven; let stand 2 minutes before removing from cookie sheet. Place on wire rack and cool completely. Repeat with remaining cookie dough.

Calories 160
  Calories from fat 65
Total fat 7.0 g
  Saturated fat 0.6 g
  Trans fat 0.0 g

Cholesterol 0 mg
Sodium 75 mg
Total carbohydrate 22 g
  Dietary fiber 2 g
  Sugars 8 g
Protein 3 g

EXCHANGES PER SERVING
1½ carbohydrate
1 fat

ALMOND CHERRY BISCOTTI WITH CITRUS

YIELD 12 servings | **SERVING SIZE** 2 biscotti

Italian for "biscuits," biscotti are twice baked for extra crispiness. The cherries and nuts in this recipe diversify the textures. Enjoy the biscotti with hot coffee, spiced hot tea, or as Italians would do, with vin santo dessert wine after dinner.

1/3 cup canola oil

2/3 cup sugar

1 teaspoon baking powder

1/2 teaspoon baking soda

2 large eggs

2 tablespoons lemon or orange zest

2 1/2 cups white whole-wheat flour, spooned into measuring cups and leveled

1/2 cup dried cherries

1/2 cup (2 ounces) slivered almonds, toasted

Canola oil cooking spray

1 Preheat oven to 375°F.

2 With a mixer, beat canola oil, sugar, baking powder, and baking soda on medium speed until combined. Beat in eggs and zest. Reduce to low speed, gradually adding flour, and beat to a coarse meal texture. (Dough will be fairly dry at this point.) Add cherries and almonds. Using a spoon, blend thoroughly. Knead slightly and shape into two logs 9 inches long, 1/2 inch high, and 2 inches wide. Coat a large nonstick baking sheet with cooking spray and place logs on baking sheet.

3 Bake for 18 minutes or until a wooden pick inserted in the center comes out clean. Cool on the baking sheet 20 minutes. Gently remove and place on a cutting board.

4 Reduce heat to 325°F. Using a serrated knife, carefully cut each roll crosswise into 12 slices diagonally. Place slices cut-side down on cookie sheet and bake 9 minutes on each side or until crisp and light brown. Place baking sheet on a wire rack and cool completely.

Calories 260
Calories from fat 90
Total fat 10.0 g
  Saturated fat 1.0 g
  Trans fat 0.0 g

Cholesterol 35 mg
Sodium 95 mg
Total carbohydrate 38 g
  Dietary fiber 4 g
  Sugars 16 g
Protein 5 g

EXCHANGES PER SERVING
2 1/2 carbohydrate
2 fat

Flavorful tip Let the biscotti stand for 4 hours so flavors can blend. Store in an airtight container at room temperature for up to 3 days or wrap in plastic wrap and freeze. Dried cranberries can be substituted for dried cherries and pistachios for almonds.

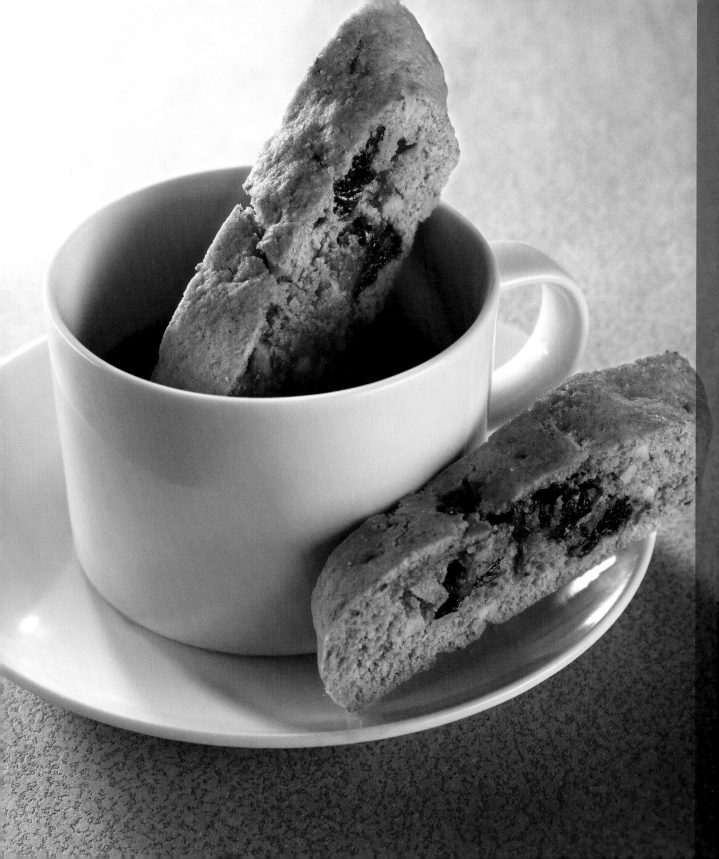

SAUTÉED APPLE-RAISIN OATMEAL

YIELD 4 servings | **SERVING SIZE** ¾ cup oatmeal

Oatmeal is a good source of fiber and the topping in this recipe is mouthwatering.

OATMEAL

- 3 cups water
- 1½ cups uncooked quick-cooking oats
- 2 tablespoons wheat bran
- ⅛ teaspoon salt

TOPPING

- ¼ cup (1 ounce) chopped pecans
- 1 tablespoon canola oil
- 1 medium-large Granny Smith apple (about 6 ounces), halved, cored, and chopped
- ¼ cup raisins
- ½ teaspoon ground cinnamon
- ¼ teaspoon ground nutmeg
- 1 teaspoon vanilla extract
- 2 tablespoons maple syrup or honey

1 Bring water to a boil over high heat in a medium saucepan; stir in oats, wheat bran, and salt. Return just to a boil, reduce heat, and simmer uncovered 6 minutes or until thickened.

2 Meanwhile, heat a medium nonstick skillet over medium-high heat. Add pecans and cook 2 minutes or until lightly browned. Remove from skillet and set aside on a separate plate. Heat canola oil in the skillet and add apple, raisins, cinnamon, and nutmeg. Cook 3 minutes or until very tender. Remove from heat and add vanilla and nuts.

3 To serve, spoon equal amounts of oatmeal into four bowls, drizzle syrup evenly over each serving, and spoon equal amounts of apple mixture in center.

		EXCHANGES PER SERVING	
Calories 280	Cholesterol 0 mg		
Calories from fat 100	Sodium 80 mg	1½ starch	*Flavorful tip* Cooking the apple in a small amount of canola oil softens its texture and flavors.
Total fat 11.0 g	Total carbohydrate 42 g	1 fruit	
Saturated fat 1.1 g	Dietary fiber 6 g	2 fat	
Trans fat 0.0 g	Sugars 17 g		
	Protein 5 g		

CREAMY APRICOT-MANGO SMOOTHIES

YIELD 4 servings | **SERVING SIZE** ¾ cup

For breakfast on the run or simply after a run, try these nutritious and delicious smoothies. Including canola oil ties all of the flavors together while giving the smoothies a rich texture.

2 cups fresh or frozen mango slices
1 cup frozen fruit, such as strawberries
½ cup nonfat vanilla yogurt
½ cup ice cubes
½ cup apricot nectar
½ cup white grape juice
2 tablespoons fresh lime juice
2 tablespoons canola oil

1 Combine all ingredients in a blender, secure the lid, and purée until smooth. Serve immediately for peak flavors and texture.

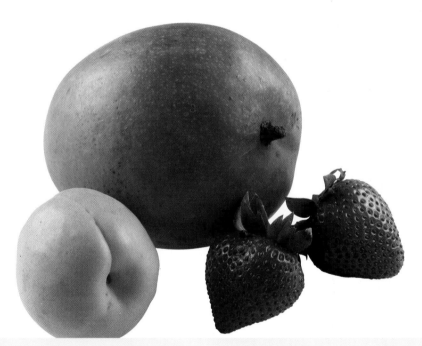

Fresh tip Peaches or seasonal fruit may be substituted for mango. Experiment to create your own signature smoothie.

Calories 180
  Calories from fat 65
Total fat 7.0 g
  Saturated fat 0.6 g
  Trans fat 0.0 g

Cholesterol 0 mg
Sodium 20 mg
Total carbohydrate 29 g
  Dietary fiber 3 g
  Sugars 23 g
Protein 2 g

EXCHANGES PER SERVING
2 fruit
1½ fat

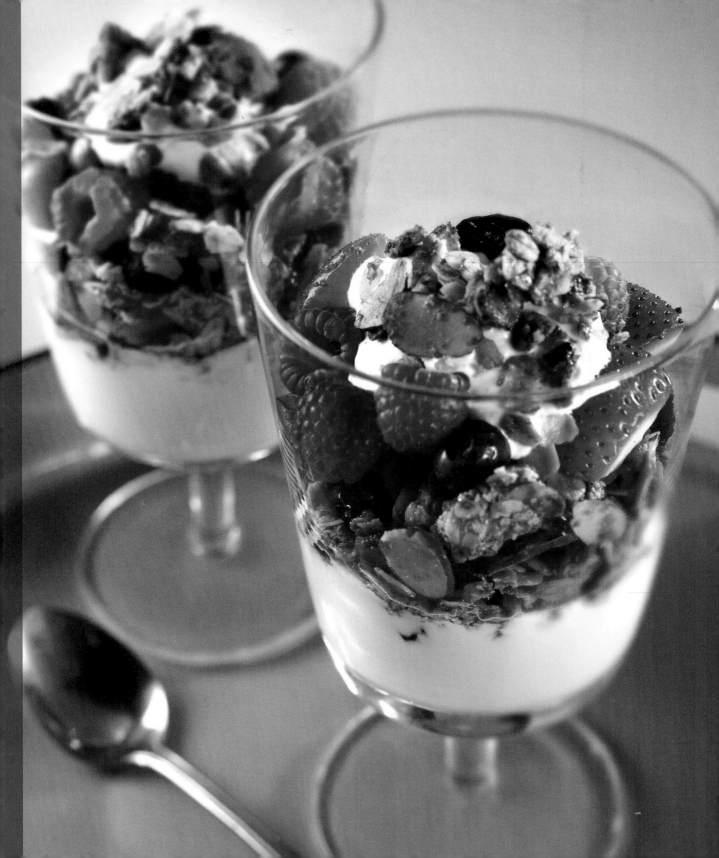

CANOLA GRANOLA

YIELD 12 servings | **SERVING SIZE** ⅓ cup

Fill several small snack bags with this healthy granola to have on hand when you need a quick pick-me-up or layer it with yogurt and fresh fruit to create a striking parfait.

Canola oil cooking spray

2 cups rolled oats

⅓ cup wheat germ

½ cup (2 ounces) almond slices

2 teaspoons ground cinnamon

¼ teaspoon plus ⅛ teaspoon salt, divided

¼ cup canola oil

¼ cup maple syrup

1 tablespoon fat-free milk

2 teaspoons vanilla extract

1 cup dried cherries

1 tablespoon orange zest

1 Preheat oven to 300°F. Coat a baking sheet with cooking spray.

2 Combine oats, wheat germ, almonds, cinnamon, and ¼ teaspoon salt in a large bowl. Add canola oil, syrup, milk, and vanilla, stirring constantly.

3 Spread mixture on a baking sheet in a layer about ¼ inch thick. Bake 25–30 minutes until browned, stirring two or three times during cooking while breaking up large pieces. Remove from the oven, sprinkle evenly with remaining ⅛ teaspoon salt, cherries, and zest. Cool completely. Store in an airtight container in the refrigerator for up to 2 weeks.

Fresh tip Serve ⅓ cup granola over 6 ounces nonfat vanilla yogurt sweetened with a sugar substitute and ½ cup quartered strawberries and you'll get 9 grams of protein, 4 grams of fiber, vitamin C, calcium, and more!

GRANOLA
Calories 200
  Calories from fat 70
Total fat 8.0 g
  Saturated fat 0.7 g
  Trans fat 0.0 g

Cholesterol 0 mg
Sodium 80 mg
Total carbohydrate 29 g
  Dietary fiber 3 g
  Sugars 15 g
Protein 4 g

GRANOLA EXCHANGES PER SERVING
2 carbohydrate
1½ fat

PARFAIT
Calories 285
  Calories from fat 80
Total fat 9.0 g
  Saturated fat 0.8 g
  Trans fat 0.0 g

Cholesterol 5 mg
Sodium 160 mg
Total carbohydrate 45 g
  Dietary fiber 5 g
  Sugars 26 g
Protein 9 g

PARFAIT EXCHANGES PER SERVING
½ fat-free milk
2½ carbohydrate
1½ fat

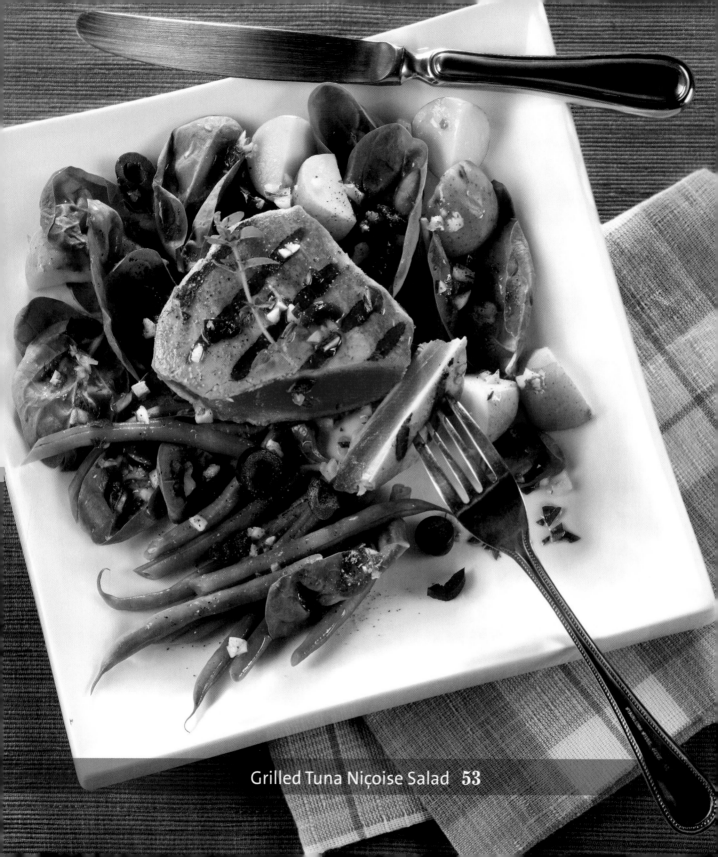

Grilled Tuna Niçoise Salad 53

LUNCH

Corn and Skillet-Roasted Poblano Soup | 44

Ham and Lentil Soup with Cloves | 45

Hearty Minestrone with Sausage | 46

Garlic White Bean Soup with
   Smoked Sausage | 47

Creamy Pumpkin-Apple Bisque | 48

Vegetable Penne Salad with Feta | 50

Bulgur and Rosemary-Edamame Salad | 51

Black Bean, Jalapeño, and Yellow Rice
   Salad | 52

Grilled Tuna Niçoise Salad | 53

Crunchy Chicken-Cilantro Lettuce Wraps | 55

Spring Greens with Chicken and Sweet
   Pomegranate Vinaigrette | 56

Greek Pepperoncini Pitas | 57

Cajun Pile-Ups with Pepper Sauce | 58

Italian-Style Sub with Dijon-Garlic Spread | 60

Turkey-Swiss Panini | 61

Vegetarian Sandwich with Sun-Dried
   Tomato Spread | 62

Open-Faced Sloppy Joes | 64

Lentil Tortillas | 65

CORN AND SKILLET-ROASTED POBLANO SOUP

YIELD 4 servings | **SERVING SIZE** 1 cup

This hearty and spicy soup will warm your core and make you want more.

1 tablespoon canola oil

3 medium poblano peppers, chopped (2 cups)

1 cup chopped onions

2 cups frozen corn kernels, thawed

1 can (14 ounces) reduced-sodium chicken broth

1½ ounces light cream cheese, soft tub variety

¾ cup fat-free milk

1 container (4 ounces) diced pimiento, drained

½ teaspoon ground cumin

¼ teaspoon salt

1½ ounces shredded reduced-fat sharp cheddar cheese

¼ cup chopped fresh cilantro leaves

1 Heat canola oil in a Dutch oven over medium-high heat. Add poblano peppers, onions, and corn. Cook 6 minutes or until just beginning to richly brown, stirring frequently. Add broth and bring to a boil over medium-high heat; then reduce heat, cover, and simmer 5 minutes.

2 Place ½ cup of pepper mixture and cream cheese in a blender, secure lid, and purée until smooth. Return puréed mixture to Dutch oven; add milk, pimiento, cumin, and salt. Cook 2 minutes to heat thoroughly.

3 To serve, spoon equal amounts of soup into four shallow bowls and top with equal amounts of cheese and cilantro.

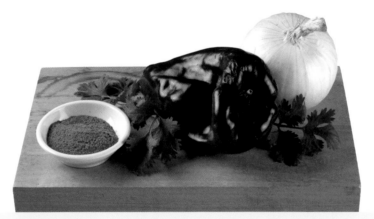

		EXCHANGES PER SERVING	
Calories 215	Cholesterol 15 mg		
Calories from fat 80	Sodium 600 mg		
Total fat 9.0 g	Total carbohydrate 29 g	1 starch	
Saturated fat 2.9 g	Dietary fiber 4 g	3 vegetable	
Trans fat 0.0 g	Sugars 12 g	1½ fat	
	Protein 10 g		

Flavorful tip Poblano peppers are dark green and heart-shaped, ranging in heat from mild to medium. The darker the pepper, the richer the flavor. For a spicier dish, use some of the chile pepper seeds.

HAM AND LENTIL SOUP
with Cloves

YIELD 4 servings | **SERVING SIZE** 1½ cups

This unique twist on bean and ham soup has a subtle sweetness due to the cloves. Just a few cloves are enough to enhance the flavor profile.

2 tablespoons canola oil, divided

1½ cups (6 ounces) extra-lean diced ham

1 cup thinly sliced carrots

1½ cups chopped onions

¾ cup thinly sliced celery

2 cloves garlic, minced

1 can (14 ounces) reduced-sodium chicken broth

2½ cups water

1 cup (6 ounces) dried brown lentils, rinsed

½ teaspoon dried thyme leaves

2 dried bay leaves

3 whole cloves

¼ teaspoon black pepper

¼ teaspoon salt

1 Heat 1 teaspoon canola oil in a Dutch oven over medium-high heat. Tilt pan to coat bottom lightly, then add ham and brown, stirring frequently. Set aside on a separate plate.

2 Heat remaining 1 tablespoon plus 2 teaspoons canola oil in a Dutch oven. Add carrots, onions, and celery, and cook 5 minutes or until beginning to richly brown on edges, stirring frequently. Add garlic and cook 15 seconds. Add broth, water, lentils, thyme, bay leaves, cloves, and black pepper. Increase heat to high, bring to a boil, reduce heat, cover tightly, and simmer 30 minutes or until lentils are soft.

3 Remove from heat and stir in ham and salt. To serve, spoon equal amounts of soup into four shallow bowls.

Fast tip Lean ham usually contains water, so using a very small amount of canola oil when browning the ham will prevent it from spattering.

Calories 295	Cholesterol 20 mg	**EXCHANGES PER SERVING**
Calories from fat 80	Sodium 880 mg	1½ starch
Total fat 9.0 g	Total carbohydrate 34 g	1 vegetable
Saturated fat 0.9 g	Dietary fiber 11 g	2 lean meat
Trans fat 0.0 g	Sugars 7 g	1 fat
	Protein 21 g	

HEARTY MINESTRONE WITH SAUSAGE

YIELD 6 servings | **SERVING SIZE** 1 cup

This chunky soup has a rich flavor from browned sausage. Using a small amount of a higher fat ingredient like sausage adds great flavor while keeping calories in check.

3 teaspoons canola oil, divided

½ of 8-ounce package reduced-fat breakfast sausage

4 ounces sliced mushrooms

1 medium zucchini, thinly sliced

1 cup chopped green bell pepper

1 can (14.5 ounces) stewed tomatoes with Italian seasonings

2 cups water

⅛ teaspoon dried red pepper flakes (optional)

¼ of 13.25-ounce package (3 ounces) dry multigrain vermicelli noodles, broken into thirds

2 cups (about 1 ounce) loosely packed baby spinach

⅓ cup chopped fresh basil leaves

1 tablespoon cider vinegar

½ teaspoon sugar

¼ teaspoon salt

2 tablespoons grated Parmesan cheese (optional)

1 Heat 1 teaspoon canola oil in a Dutch oven over medium-high heat. Add sausage and cook until browned, stirring constantly. Remove sausage from Dutch oven; set aside on a separate plate.

2 Heat remaining 2 teaspoons canola oil in a Dutch oven. Add mushrooms, zucchini, and bell pepper; cook 2 minutes, stirring constantly. Add tomatoes, water, and pepper flakes. Bring to a boil over high heat, reduce heat, cover, and simmer 15 minutes or until tomatoes are very tender. Break up large pieces of tomato with a spoon.

3 Meanwhile, cook pasta in a separate pot according to package directions, omitting any salt or fat. Drain well.

4 Remove soup from heat and add remaining ingredients, except pasta and Parmesan.

5 To serve, spoon equal amounts of soup into six shallow bowls, mound equal amounts of pasta in the center of each bowl, and sprinkle evenly with Parmesan.

		EXCHANGES PER SERVING	
Calories 145	Cholesterol 10 mg		
Calories from fat 55	Sodium 395 mg	½ starch	
Total fat 6.0 g	Total carbohydrate 18 g	2 vegetable	
Saturated fat 1.2 g	Dietary fiber 4 g	1 fat	
Trans fat 0.0 g	Sugars 5 g		
	Protein 7 g		

Fast tip To make this soup ahead of time but retain a fresh taste, cook it for 15 minutes and make the pasta separately. Then cool and refrigerate the soup and pasta. To serve, reheat both, combine, and top with Parmesan.

GARLIC WHITE BEAN SOUP
with Smoked Sausage

YIELD 4 servings | **SERVING SIZE** 1 cup

This hearty, smoky soup is ready to serve in less than 30 minutes. It's perfect on a cold and rainy day!

1½ tablespoons canola oil, divided

1½ cups (6 ounces) smoked turkey sausage, diced

1½ cups chopped onions

1 cup matchstick carrots

4 medium cloves garlic, minced

1 can (15 ounces) no-salt-added navy beans, rinsed and drained

1 can (14 ounces) reduced-sodium chicken broth

1 cup water

1 teaspoon dried oregano leaves, crumbled

½ teaspoon dried thyme leaves, crumbled

1 teaspoon Worcestershire sauce

¾ teaspoon black pepper

1 tablespoon liquid smoke

1 Heat 1½ teaspoons canola oil in a Dutch oven over medium-high heat. Add sausage and cook until browned, about 2 minutes. Remove sausage from Dutch oven; set aside on a separate plate.

2 Add remaining 1 tablespoon canola oil and reduce to medium heat. Add onions and carrots; cook 3 minutes or until onions are translucent, stirring frequently. Add garlic; cook 15 seconds. Add remaining ingredients, except liquid smoke and sausage. Bring to a boil over high heat, reduce heat, cover, and simmer 20 minutes or until onions are tender.

3 Remove from heat and add liquid smoke and sausage. Cover and let stand 10 minutes. To serve, spoon equal amounts of soup into four shallow bowls.

Flavorful tip Allow the soup to stand 10 minutes so its flavors can absorb. It is important to add the sausage at the end of the cooking time; otherwise, the rich, smoky flavors will break down and become lost.

Calories 265	Cholesterol 30 mg	**EXCHANGES PER SERVING**	
Calories from fat 90	Sodium 665 mg	1 starch	
Total fat 10.0 g	Total carbohydrate 30 g	2 vegetable	
Saturated fat 1.9 g	Dietary fiber 8 g	1 lean meat	
Trans fat 0.0 g	Sugars 5 g	1½ fat	
	Protein 14 g		

CREAMY PUMPKIN-APPLE BISQUE

YIELD 4 servings | **SERVING SIZE** 1 cup

Curl up by the fire and enjoy the taste of fall with this decadent soup.

- 1 tablespoon canola oil
- 1 cup diced onions
- ½ medium Gala apple, peeled and chopped
- 1 can (14 ounces) reduced-sodium chicken broth
- ½ of 15-ounce can solid pumpkin
- 2 tablespoons sugar
- 1½ teaspoons ground cinnamon
- ½ teaspoon ground cumin
- ½ teaspoon salt
- ⅛ teaspoon cayenne pepper
- 1½ cups fat-free half and half
- ¼ cup fat-free sour cream

1 Heat canola oil in a large saucepan over medium-high heat. Add onions and apple; cook 5 minutes or until onions begin to brown.

2 Place onion mixture in a blender with 1 cup broth. Secure lid and purée until smooth. Return onion mixture to saucepan; add remaining ingredients, except half and half and sour cream. Bring to boil over high heat, reduce heat, cover tightly, and simmer 15 minutes.

3 Remove from heat and gradually add half and half while stirring. To serve, spoon equal amounts of soup into four shallow bowls and top with dollops of sour cream.

Calories 175
  Calories from fat 45
Total fat 5.0 g
  Saturated fat 1.1 g
  Trans fat 0.0 g
Cholesterol 5 mg
Sodium 635 mg
Total carbohydrate 26 g
  Dietary fiber 3 g
  Sugars 17 g
Protein 6 g

EXCHANGES PER SERVING
2 carbohydrate
1 fat

Flavorful tip Adding the apple while browning the onion brings out the sugars of the apple and richly browns the onions quickly.

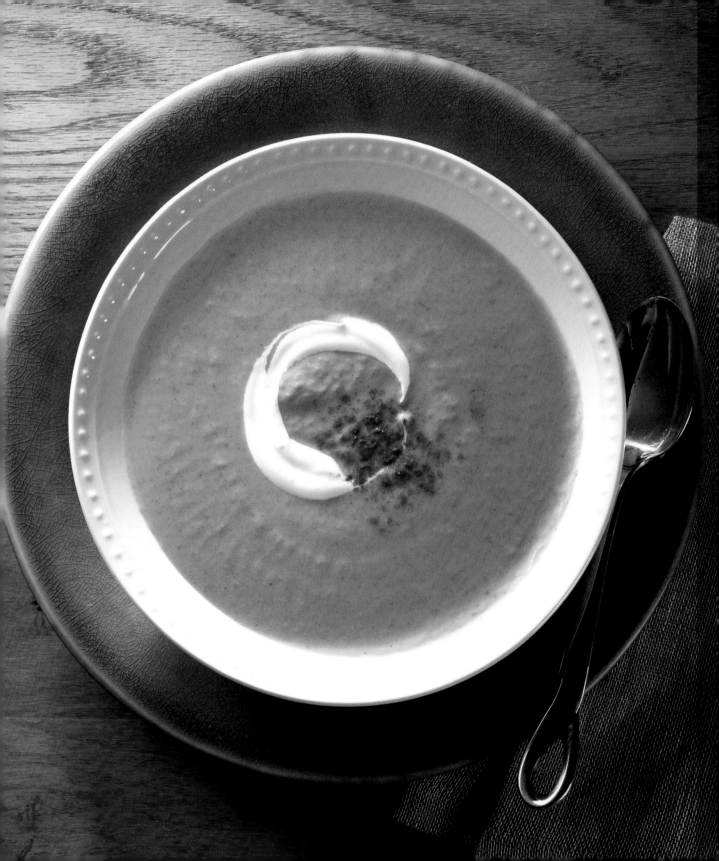

VEGETABLE PENNE SALAD WITH FETA

YIELD 4 servings | **SERVING SIZE** 1½ cups

This eye-catching pasta salad entices with its black beans, red peppers, yellow squash, and green parsley.

SALAD

- 1 cup (4 ounces) dry whole-grain penne or rotini pasta
- 1 can (13.75 ounces) quartered artichoke hearts, drained
- ½ of 15-ounce can no-salt-added black beans, rinsed and drained
- ½ medium red bell pepper, cut into thin, 2-inch-long pieces
- 1 small yellow squash, halved lengthwise and thinly sliced
- ¾ cup (3 ounces) reduced-fat feta cheese, crumbled

VINAIGRETTE

- ⅓ cup chopped fresh parsley leaves
- 2 tablespoons canola oil
- 3 tablespoons cider vinegar
- 1 tablespoon dried oregano leaves
- 1 teaspoon dried rosemary leaves
- 2 medium cloves garlic, minced

1 Cook pasta according to package directions, omitting any salt or fat.

2 Meanwhile, prepare vegetables and make vinaigrette. Drain pasta in colander and run under cold water to completely cool. Combine salad ingredients, except feta, in a large bowl. Pour vinaigrette over pasta mixture. Toss gently, yet thoroughly, until well blended. Add feta and toss gently.

3 Let stand 30 minutes before serving to absorb flavors.

		EXCHANGES PER SERVING
Calories 300	Cholesterol 5 mg	
Calories from fat 100	Sodium 475 mg	2 starch
Total fat 11.0 g	Total carbohydrate 40 g	1 vegetable
Saturated fat 2.6 g	Dietary fiber 8 g	1 lean meat
Trans fat 0.0 g	Sugars 5 g	1½ fat
	Protein 13 g	

Flavorful tip Making your own vinaigrette allows you to control the fat and flavor. Canola oil is the perfect base due to its low saturated fat content, light texture, and neutral taste, which lets the flavors of the seasonings shine.

BULGUR AND ROSEMARY-EDAMAME SALAD

YIELD 4 servings | **SERVING SIZE** 1 cup

Full of lemon and fresh herb flavors, this salad is perfect for your next patio party.

2 cups water

½ cup quick-cooking bulgur

1 cup diced pre-cooked chicken breast

1 cup frozen shelled edamame, thawed

1 cup (½ ounce) loosely packed baby spinach, coarsely chopped

½ cup chopped fresh mint leaves

¼ cup chopped fresh parsley leaves

1 tablespoon grated lemon zest

2–3 tablespoons lemon juice

2 tablespoons canola oil

1 teaspoon chopped fresh rosemary leaves or ¼ teaspoon dried rosemary leaves, crumbled

½ teaspoon salt

1 Bring water to a boil in a medium saucepan over high heat. Add bulgur, reduce heat, cover tightly, and simmer 10 minutes or until water is absorbed.

2 Meanwhile, combine remaining ingredients in a medium bowl.

3 Place bulgur in a fine-mesh strainer and run under cold water to completely cool. Drain well; stir into chicken mixture. Toss gently, yet thoroughly, to blend.

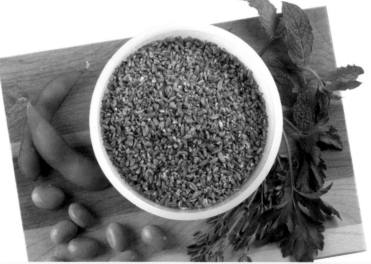

Calories 220
Calories from fat 100
Total fat 11.0 g
Saturated fat 1.2 g
Trans fat 0.0 g

Cholesterol 30 mg
Sodium 330 mg
Total carbohydrate 15 g
Dietary fiber 5 g
Sugars 1 g
Protein 17 g

EXCHANGES PER SERVING
1 starch
2 lean meat
1 fat

BLACK BEAN, JALAPEÑO, AND YELLOW RICE SALAD

YIELD 4 servings | **SERVING SIZE** 1½ cups

This dish visually connotes health and freshness. Chopped, pickled jalapeño spreads the heat evenly while giving a new twist on flavor.

1½ cups water

¾ cup quick-cooking brown rice

¼ teaspoon ground turmeric

1 can (15 ounces) black beans, rinsed and drained

1 cup grape tomatoes, quartered

½ medium unpeeled cucumber, seeded and chopped

½ cup (2 ounces) mozzarella, cut into ¼-inch cubes

2 tablespoons chopped fresh cilantro leaves

1–2 tablespoons chopped pickled jalapeño pepper slices (about 4–8 slices)

2 tablespoons fresh lime juice

1 medium clove garlic, minced

2 tablespoons canola oil

½ teaspoon salt

1 Bring water to a boil in a medium saucepan. Add rice and turmeric; return to a boil, reduce heat, cover tightly, and simmer 10 minutes or until water is absorbed.

2 Meanwhile, combine remaining ingredients in a large bowl.

3 Place rice on a sheet of foil or baking sheet in a thin layer to cool quickly, about 10 minutes. Add rice to bean mixture; toss gently, yet thoroughly, to blend. Serve immediately for peak flavors.

Calories 320
  Calories from fat 90
Total fat 10.0 g
  Saturated fat 2.1 g
  Trans fat 0.0 g

Cholesterol 10 mg
Sodium 490 mg
Total carbohydrate 45 g
  Dietary fiber 8 g
  Sugars 4 g
Protein 12 g

EXCHANGES PER SERVING

3 starch
1 lean meat
1 fat

GRILLED TUNA NIÇOISE SALAD

YIELD 4 servings | **SERVING SIZE** 1½ cups salad + 1 tuna steak

This light dish is a great choice for a summer luncheon or al fresco dinner.

SALAD

- ¾ lb small red potatoes, diced
- ½ lb green beans, trimmed
- 4 tuna steaks (4 ounces each, about ¾-inch thick)
  Canola oil cooking spray
- 4 cups (2 ounces) baby spinach leaves
- 16 pitted kalamata olives, coarsely chopped

VINAIGRETTE

- 2 tablespoons canola oil
- 2 tablespoons red wine vinegar
- 1 tablespoon water
- ⅛ teaspoon salt
- ½ medium clove garlic, minced
- ⅛ teaspoon dried red pepper flakes
- 1 tablespoon chopped fresh oregano leaves or 1 teaspoon dried oregano leaves

1 Steam potatoes and green beans 6 minutes or just until tender. Drain and rinse with cold water, shaking off excess liquid.

2 While vegetables cook, combine vinaigrette ingredients in a small jar, secure with lid, and shake well to blend completely. Set aside ¼ cup vinaigrette and brush remaining vinaigrette (1 tablespoon) over fish.

3 Coat a grill pan with cooking spray and heat over medium-high heat until hot. Grill tuna over high heat 3 minutes on each side or until medium-rare or desired degree of doneness. (Do not overcook or fish will be tough.)

4 Divide greens equally on four serving plates. Arrange potatoes, green beans, and olives over greens. Drizzle 1 tablespoon vinaigrette evenly over each salad and top with tuna.

Fresh tip Fish is always best if purchased and prepared the same day.

Calories 345	Cholesterol 40 mg
Calories from fat 125	Sodium 280 mg
Total fat 14.0 g	Total carbohydrate 26 g
Saturated fat 2.2 g	Dietary fiber 5 g
Trans fat 0.0 g	Sugars 2 g
	Protein 29 g

EXCHANGES PER SERVING

1½ starch
1 vegetable
3 lean meat
1½ fat

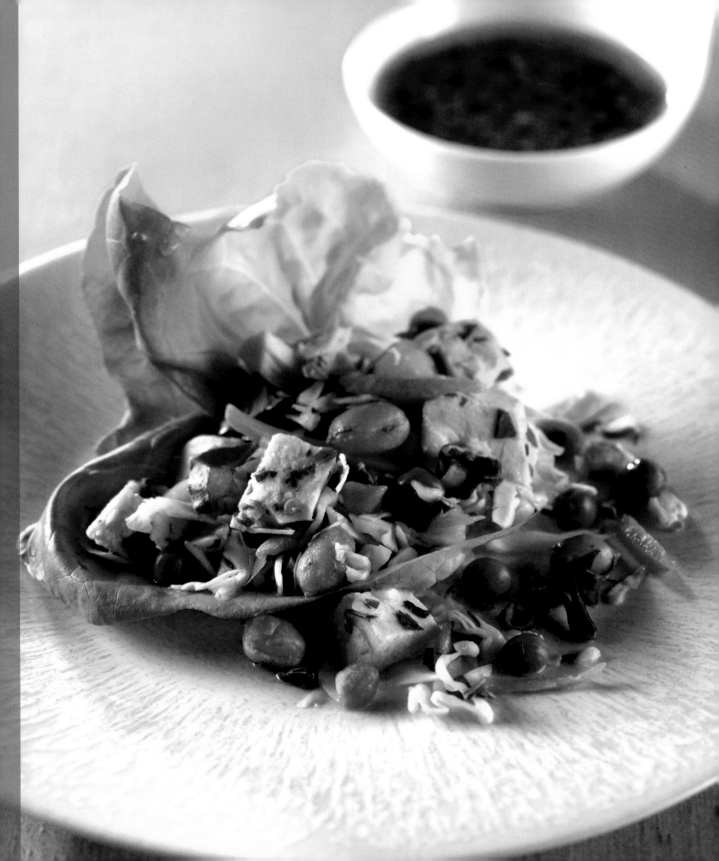

CRUNCHY CHICKEN-CILANTRO LETTUCE WRAPS

YIELD 4 servings | **SERVING SIZE** 3 lettuce wraps

Lettuce wraps look fun and festive, especially when they're arranged on a large platter.

SAUCE

- 3 tablespoons reduced-sodium soy sauce
- 2 tablespoons sugar
- 2 tablespoons fresh lime juice
- 1 tablespoon canola oil
- 1 tablespoon water
- 1–1½ teaspoons orange zest
- ¼ teaspoon dried red pepper flakes

FILLING

- 2 cups bagged coleslaw mix
- ½ of 8-ounce can sliced water chestnuts, drained and cut in half
- ½ cup frozen green peas, thawed
- 1 cup pre-cooked diced chicken breast
- ⅓ cup (1½ ounces) dry roasted peanuts, toasted
- ¼ cup chopped fresh cilantro leaves
- 12 large Boston Bibb or romaine lettuce leaves, rinsed and patted dry

1 Combine sauce ingredients in a small bowl and whisk until well blended. Combine filling ingredients in a medium bowl.

2 To serve, arrange three lettuce leaves on each of four dinner plates and spoon equal amounts of filling on top. Serve with sauce on side. Have people roll up their own lettuce wraps and dip into sauce.

Flavorful tip The canola oil in the dipping sauce helps the sauce adhere slightly to the lettuce.

Calories 225	Cholesterol 30 mg
Calories from fat 90	Sodium 585 mg
Total fat 10.0 g	Total carbohydrate 17 g
Saturated fat 1.4 g	Dietary fiber 4 g
Trans fat 0.0 g	Sugars 10 g
	Protein 16 g

EXCHANGES PER SERVING

1 carbohydrate
2 lean meat
1½ fat

SPRING GREENS WITH CHICKEN
and Sweet Pomegranate Vinaigrette

YIELD 4 servings | **SERVING SIZE** 1½ cups

The fruity vinaigrette makes the greens and chicken dance on the plate.

VINAIGRETTE

- ¼ cup pomegranate juice
- 2 tablespoons white balsamic vinegar
- 1 tablespoon plus 2 teaspoons canola oil
- 1 tablespoon pourable sugar substitute
- 1 teaspoon orange zest
- ¼ teaspoon salt
- ⅛ teaspoon dried red pepper flakes

SALAD

- 1 teaspoon canola oil
- 2 boneless chicken breasts (¾ lb total), rinsed and patted dry
- 1 teaspoon coarsely ground black pepper
- 1 bag (5 ounces) spring greens
- ½ of 14.5-ounce can beet slices, rinsed, drained, and halved
- ½ cup thinly sliced red onion
- ⅓ cup (1½ ounces) crumbled reduced-fat blue cheese

1 Combine all vinaigrette ingredients, except 1 teaspoon canola oil, in a jar, secure lid, and shake until well blended.

2 Heat remaining 1 teaspoon canola oil in a medium nonstick skillet and tilt to coat bottom lightly. Sprinkle both sides of chicken with black pepper and cook 5 minutes on each side or until juices run clear and it is no longer pink in the center. Set aside on cutting board. Let stand 3 minutes before slicing.

3 Arrange equal amounts of salad greens on four dinner plates. Top with beet halves and onion. Spoon vinaigrette evenly over all. Arrange equal amounts of chicken on top and sprinkle with blue cheese. Serve immediately for peak flavors and texture.

Calories 225
　Calories from fat 100
Total fat 11.0 g
　Saturated fat 2.4 g
　Trans fat 0.0 g

Cholesterol 55 mg
Sodium 410 mg
Total carbohydrate 9 g
　Dietary fiber 1 g
　Sugars 7 g
Protein 22 g

EXCHANGES PER SERVING
1 vegetable
3 lean meat
1½ fat

Flavorful tip Cranberry juice may be substituted for pomegranate in the vinaigrette, which may be made up to 48 hours in advance.

GREEK PEPPERONCINI PITAS

Pepperoncini peppers are traditionally used in antipasto, but adding them to sandwiches and salads provides a new dimension of flavor.

VINAIGRETTE

2 tablespoons canola oil

2 tablespoons cider vinegar

2 tablespoons dry white wine

1 teaspoon dried oregano leaves

FILLING

3 cups (3 ounces) loosely packed chopped romaine

1/2 cup quartered grape tomatoes

1/2 cup finely chopped green bell pepper

6 pepperoncini peppers, chopped (1.5 ounces)

16 slices (about 1 ounce) turkey pepperoni, halved

4 whole-grain pita rounds, cut in half crosswise, warmed

1/2 cup (2 ounces) crumbled reduced-fat feta cheese

1 Combine vinaigrette ingredients in a small bowl and whisk until well blended.

2 Combine romaine, tomatoes, bell pepper, pepperoncini peppers, and pepperoni in a medium bowl. Pour vinaigrette over all and toss gently, yet thoroughly, to coat well. Place equal amounts of romaine mixture in each of the warmed pita halves; sprinkle evenly with feta.

Fresh tip For even more protein and slightly less sodium, substitute turkey pepperoni with 1 cup of chopped, cooked chicken breast. For variety, serve this dish as a main salad by omitting the pitas and serving each salad with a slice of whole-wheat bread.

		EXCHANGES PER SERVING
Calories 300	Cholesterol 15 mg	
Calories from fat 110	Sodium 705 mg	
Total fat 12.0 g	Total carbohydrate 40 g	2 starch
Saturated fat 2.4 g	Dietary fiber 6 g	1 vegetable
Trans fat 0.0 g	Sugars 3 g	1 lean meat
	Protein 12 g	1 1/2 fat

CAJUN PILE-UPS
with Pepper Sauce

YIELD 4 servings | **SERVING SIZE** 2 halves

Reminiscent of New Orleans, these sandwiches are ragin' with flavor from the hot sauce and banana pepper.

SAUCE

1½ tablespoons canola oil

2 teaspoons Louisiana-style hot sauce

2 teaspoons cider vinegar

¼ teaspoon dried oregano leaves

SANDWICH

½ of 16-ounce loaf multigrain Italian bread, cut into 8 slices

4 cups (about 2 ounces) loosely packed, torn romaine pieces

2 tablespoons (1–2 ounces) pickled mild banana pepper rings, drained

1 medium tomato, cut into 4 slices and then halved

½ cup thinly sliced red onion

½ medium green bell pepper, thinly sliced

¼ lb deli-sliced lean ham

2 thin slices (1½ ounces) reduced-fat Swiss cheese, cut in half

1 Combine sauce ingredients in a small bowl and stir until completely blended.

2 Drizzle one side of each bread slice with sauce and top four bread slices (sauce side up) with equal amounts of filling ingredients in the order listed, beginning with torn lettuce. Top with remaining bread slices (sauce side down), press down slightly, and cut each sandwich in half diagonally.

		EXCHANGES PER SERVING
Calories 275	Cholesterol 20 mg	1½ starch
Calories from fat 90	Sodium 530 mg	1 vegetable
Total fat 10.0 g	Total carbohydrate 30 g	2 lean meat
Saturated fat 2.0 g	Dietary fiber 5 g	1 fat
Trans fat 0.0 g	Sugars 6 g	
	Protein 18 g	

Flavorful tip Mixing canola oil with the tangy vinegar and spicy hot sauce creates an intensely flavorful sauce...a little goes a very long way! If you're not a fan of spicy food, opt for a milder hot sauce with more flavor than heat.

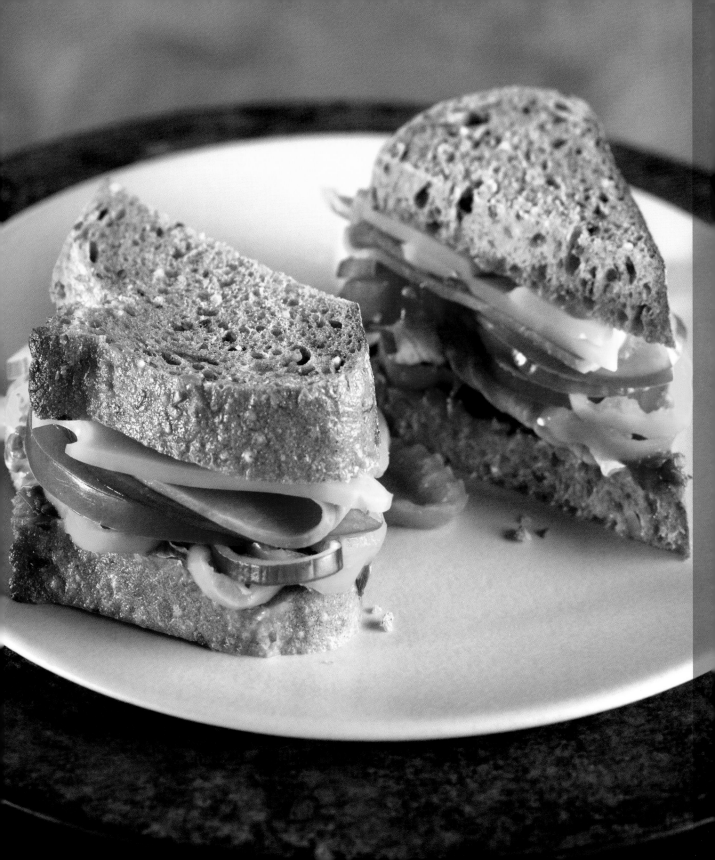

ITALIAN-STYLE SUB
with Dijon-Garlic Spread

YIELD 4 servings | **SERVING SIZE** ¼ sub

This sub includes prosciutto, which is the Italian word for "ham" that connotes aged and dry-cured ham in English. Prosciutto is seasoned and salt-cured, not smoked, and can be found in the deli section of major grocery stores.

SPREAD

- 1 tablespoon coarse-grain Dijon mustard
- 1 tablespoon canola oil
- 1 tablespoon red wine vinegar
- 2 cloves garlic, minced

SANDWICH

- ¾ of 16-ounce loaf multigrain Italian bread, cut in half lengthwise
- ¼ cup chopped fresh basil leaves
- 1 medium tomato, thinly sliced
- 4 thin slices prosciutto (2 ounces total)
- ½ cup thinly sliced green bell pepper
- 4 cups (2 ounces) loosely packed spring greens

1 Hollow out top and bottom halves of bread, leaving ½-inch-thick shell. Reserve torn bread for another use.

2 Combine spread ingredients in a small bowl. Put 1½ tablespoons of spread over cut side of each bread half. Sprinkle bottom half of loaf evenly with basil and top with tomato slices, prosciutto, bell pepper, and greens. Cover with top half of loaf. Cut filled loaf crosswise into four equal pieces.

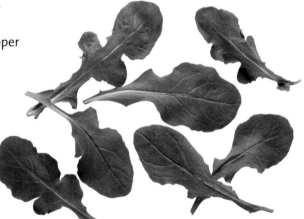

		EXCHANGES PER SERVING	
Calories 235	Cholesterol 10 mg		*Flavorful tip* The reserved torn bread
Calories from fat 70	Sodium 590 mg	1½ starch	can be used to make fresh croutons or
Total fat 8.0 g	Total carbohydrate 29 g	1 vegetable	bread crumbs. Use the savory spread
Saturated fat 1.3 g	Dietary fiber 6 g	1 lean meat	to wake up everyday sandwiches with
Trans fat 0.0 g	Sugars 6 g	1 fat	flavor and punch.
	Protein 13 g		

TURKEY-SWISS PANINI

YIELD 4 servings | **SERVING SIZE** 1 sandwich

Although panini are usually grilled in a sandwich press, a stack of plates will have the same effect. Simply pile plates on top of the sandwiches to weigh them down while they cook.

1 tablespoon plus 1 teaspoon balsamic vinegar

5 teaspoons canola oil, divided

2 medium cloves garlic, minced

½ of 16-ounce loaf multigrain Italian bread, halved lengthwise and then each half cut into four pieces

2 medium whole green onions, finely chopped

1 cup (½ ounce) loosely packed fresh spinach leaves

¼ lb deli-sliced oven roasted turkey breast

1 medium tomato, cut into 8 slices

4 thin slices (3 ounces total) reduced-fat Swiss cheese

Canola oil cooking spray

3 cups halved strawberries

1 Combine vinegar, 4 teaspoons canola oil, and garlic in a small bowl. Stir until well blended. Drizzle one side of each bread slice with vinegar mixture and top four bread slices (oil side up) with equal amounts of filling ingredients in the order listed, beginning with green onions. Top with remaining bread slices (oil side down) and press down slightly.

2 Coat a medium nonstick skillet with cooking spray, add ½ teaspoon canola oil, tilt skillet to coat bottom lightly, and place over medium heat. Add two sandwiches, then place dinner plate and four bread plates on top of sandwiches. Cook 4 minutes, turn sandwiches, top with plates, and cook 2–3 minutes or until cheese melts.

3 Place on a serving platter, cover with foil to keep warm, and repeat with remaining ½ teaspoon canola oil and two sandwiches. Serve with strawberry halves on the side.

Flavorful tip Coating the skillet with canola oil cooking spray and using a small amount of canola oil to brown the sandwiches provides optimum moisture and flavor to the sandwiches.

Calories 335	Cholesterol 20 mg
Calories from fat 110	Sodium 585 mg
Total fat 12.0 g	Total carbohydrate 37 g
Saturated fat 2.7 g	Dietary fiber 7 g
Trans fat 0.0 g	Sugars 11 g
	Protein 22 g

EXCHANGES PER SERVING

1½ starch
½ fruit
1 vegetable
2 lean meat
1½ fat

VEGETARIAN SANDWICH
with Sun-Dried Tomato Spread

YIELD 8 servings | **SERVING SIZE** 1 wedge

This will definitely be a hit at your next picnic or patio party. It looks like a big circle of bread or "boule" on a serving platter, but it's pre-cut into wedges for guests to easily enjoy.

SPREAD

16 sun-dried tomato halves

1 cup boiling water

2 tablespoons dried basil leaves

1/3 cup capers, drained

4 medium cloves garlic, peeled

1/4 cup canola oil

1/4 cup red wine vinegar

1 round loaf (16 ounces) Tuscan-style bread, halved, creating 2 rounds

FILLING

6 thin slices (4 1/2 ounces total) reduced-fat Swiss cheese

1/2 cup thinly sliced red onion

1/2–3/4 cup thinly sliced green bell pepper

4 cups (2 ounces) loosely packed spring greens

1 Place tomatoes in a small bowl, cover with boiling water, and let stand 5 minutes to soften. Place tomatoes, 1/2 cup tomato water, and remaining spread ingredients in a blender; purée until smooth.

2 Spread half of tomato mixture evenly over bottom half of bread loaf and top with filling ingredients in the order listed, starting with cheese. Spread remaining tomato mixture on top half of bread loaf and place, spread side down, on top of lettuce. Press down firmly and cut into 8 wedges.

		EXCHANGES PER SERVING	
Calories 280	Cholesterol 5 mg		
Calories from fat 100	Sodium 680 mg	2 starch	
Total fat 11.0 g	Total carbohydrate 34 g	1 vegetable	
Saturated fat 2.2 g	Dietary fiber 3 g	1 lean meat	
Trans fat 0.0 g	Sugars 3 g	1 1/2 fat	
	Protein 11 g		

Fast tip This is a great make-ahead sandwich. The spread can also be used as a "tapenade" on crostini or whole-grain crackers.

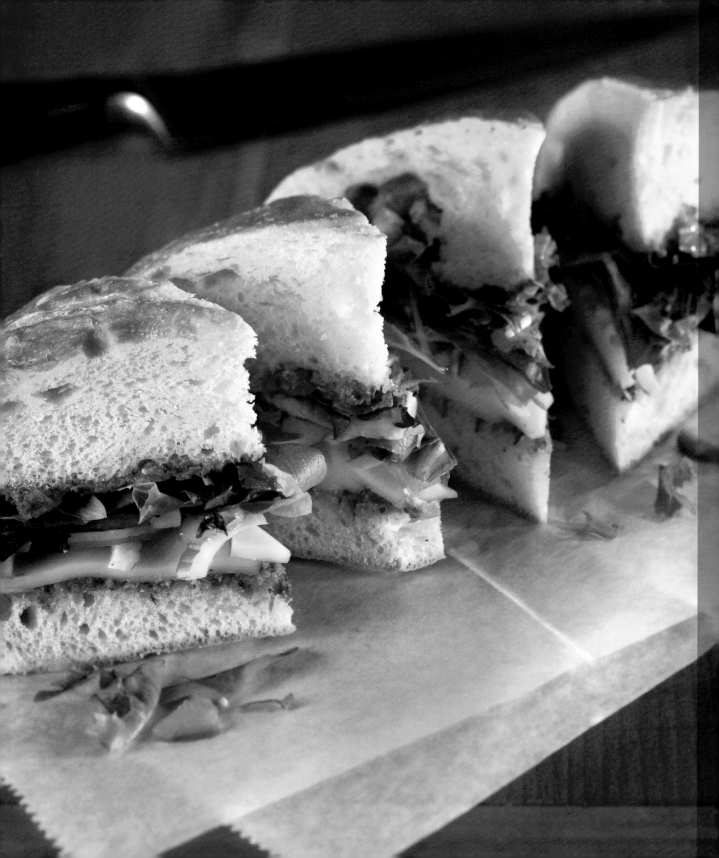

OPEN-FACED SLOPPY JOES

YIELD 4 servings | **SERVING SIZE** 2 open-faced sandwiches

Sloppy Joes always live up to their namesake. This version spills over with goodness on open-faced buns, so you get to use a fork!

1 tablespoon canola oil

¾ lb extra-lean ground turkey breast

1 medium jalapeño, thinly sliced (seeded, optional)

1 can (14.5 ounces) stewed tomatoes, Mexican-style

1 cup frozen mixed vegetables, thawed

1 teaspoon Worcestershire sauce

1 teaspoon beef bouillon granules

1 teaspoon chili powder

1 tablespoon sugar

2 teaspoons cider vinegar

1 teaspoon ground cumin

4 whole-wheat hamburger buns, split in half and toasted

1 Heat canola oil in a large nonstick skillet over medium-high heat. Cook ground turkey 2–3 minutes or until no longer pink, stirring frequently. Add jalapeño and cook 2 minutes. Add tomatoes, mixed vegetables, Worcestershire, bouillon granules, and chili powder. Bring to a boil over medium-high heat, reduce heat, cover, and simmer 15 minutes or until tomatoes are tender. Break up large pieces of tomato with the back of a spoon.

2 Add sugar, vinegar, and cumin; cook, uncovered, 5 minutes to thicken slightly. Place two bun halves on each of four dinner plates. Spoon equal amounts of turkey mixture on top of bun halves, allowing mixture to spill over sides.

		EXCHANGES PER SERVING
Calories 295	Cholesterol 40 mg	
Calories from fat 65	Sodium 840 mg	
Total fat 7.0 g	Total carbohydrate 36 g	1½ starch
Saturated fat 1.0 g	Dietary fiber 6 g	2 vegetable
Trans fat 0.0 g	Sugars 14 g	3 lean meat
	Protein 26 g	

Fast tip If desired, make four traditional Sloppy Joe sandwiches and freeze the remaining filling for later use. For variety, the Sloppy Joe mixture can be served over baked potato halves or on a bed of cooked spaghetti squash.

The taste of the Yucatan comes with every bite of these vegetarian tortillas made with green salsa, cilantro, and jalapeño.

¾ cup (4 ounces) dried brown lentils

2 cups water

½ cup salsa verde, divided

2 tablespoons canola oil, divided

½ teaspoon ground cumin

Canola oil cooking spray

8 corn tortillas, warmed

1 medium jalapeño, seeded and finely chopped

¼ cup chopped fresh cilantro leaves

½ cup (2 ounces) shredded reduced-fat Mexican blend cheese or mozzarella

2 cups loosely packed shredded lettuce

½ cup fat-free sour cream

1 Bring lentils and water to a boil in a medium saucepan over high heat; reduce heat, cover tightly and simmer 25–30 minutes or until tender. Drain in a fine-mesh strainer, place in a small bowl and add ¼ cup salsa verde, 1 tablespoon canola oil, and cumin. In a separate bowl, mix the remaining ¼ cup salsa verde and 1 tablespoon canola oil.

2 Preheat oven to 350°F. Coat a nonstick baking sheet with cooking spray. Arrange tortillas on the baking sheet and spoon equal amounts of lentil mixture on tortillas. Using the back of a spoon, spread mixture to edges of tortillas. Top with jalapeño, cilantro, and cheese. Bake 3–5 minutes or until cheese melts.

3 Place on four dinner plates and top with lettuce, sour cream, and remaining salsa verde.

Flavorful tip Adding canola oil to the salsa verde takes the edge off of the sauce, making it mellower in flavor and smoother in texture.

Calories 170
 Calories from fat 55
Total fat 6.0 g
 Saturated fat 1.2 g
 Trans fat 0.0 g

Cholesterol 5 mg
Sodium 120 mg
Total carbohydrate 21 g
 Dietary fiber 5 g
 Sugars 2 g
Protein 8 g

EXCHANGES PER SERVING
1 starch
1 lean meat
1 fat

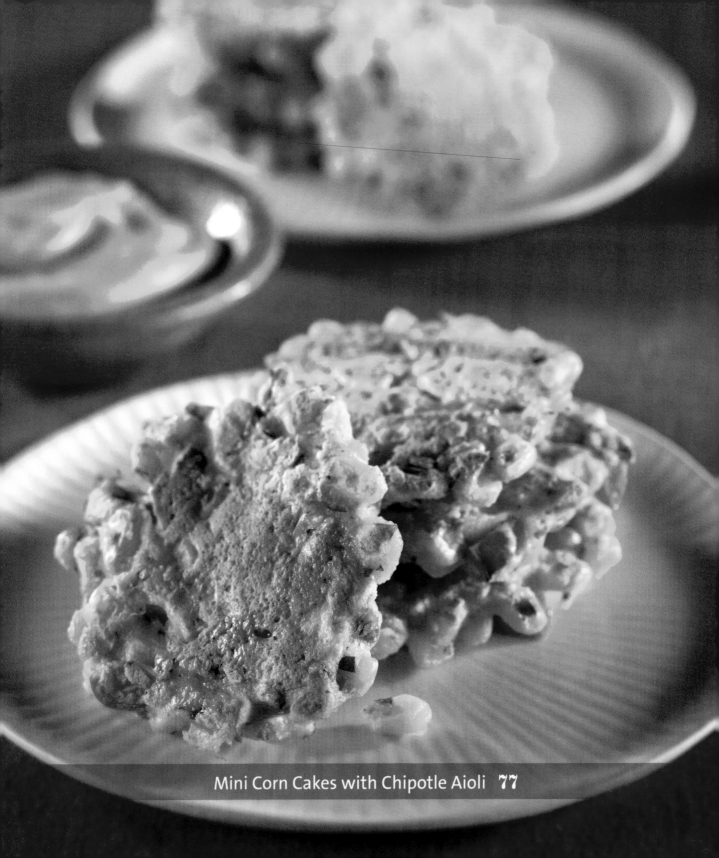

Mini Corn Cakes with Chipotle Aioli **77**

APPETIZERS

Marinated Italian Vegetable Toss | 68

Spicy Mediterranean White Bean Hummus | 70

Crunchy Red Pepper-Ginger Relish with Cucumber Rounds | 71

Creamy Black Bean Stack Dip | 73

Mini Potatoes with Caramelized Onions and Blue Cheese | 74

Soy-Marinated Mushrooms with Cilantro and Basil | 75

Crispy Baked Zucchini Spears with Lemon | 76

Mini Corn Cakes with Chipotle Aioli | 77

Basil Focaccia Wedges | 79

Mini Vegetable Panini | 80

West Indies Shrimp and Jalapeño Rounds | 81

Pork Sliders with Raspberry Mustard Sauce | 82

Mini Greek Chicken Kabobs | 84

Apricot Hoisin-Glazed Meatballs | 85

MARINATED ITALIAN VEGETABLE TOSS

YIELD 12 servings | **SERVING SIZE** ⅓ cup

This colorful vegetarian dish includes protein from chickpeas, which are nutrient-dense and popular around the world.

1 can (13.75 ounces) quartered artichoke hearts, drained

½ of 16-ounce can chickpeas, rinsed and drained

1 cup grape tomatoes

¼ cup (1 ounce) part-skim mozzarella cheese, cut into ¼-inch cubes

8 pitted kalamata olives

½ medium green bell pepper, cut into strips

2–3 tablespoons fresh oregano leaves or 1 tablespoon dried oregano leaves

1½ teaspoons chopped fresh rosemary leaves or ½ teaspoon dried rosemary leaves

2 tablespoons canola oil

1 tablespoon red wine vinegar

1 medium clove garlic, minced

⅛ teaspoon dried red pepper flakes

1 Combine all ingredients in a medium bowl and toss gently, yet thoroughly, until well coated. Serve with wooden picks or forks.

Calories 65
  Calories from fat 30
Total fat 3.5 g
  Saturated fat 0.5 g
  Trans fat 0.0 g

Cholesterol 0 mg
Sodium 140 mg
Total carbohydrate 6 g
  Dietary fiber 2 g
  Sugars 1 g
Protein 2 g

EXCHANGES PER SERVING
1 vegetable
½ fat

Fast tip In addition to bringing out ingredient flavors, canola oil binds the herbs to the vegetables. Double the recipe and use leftovers as a topping for a luncheon pasta or green salad.

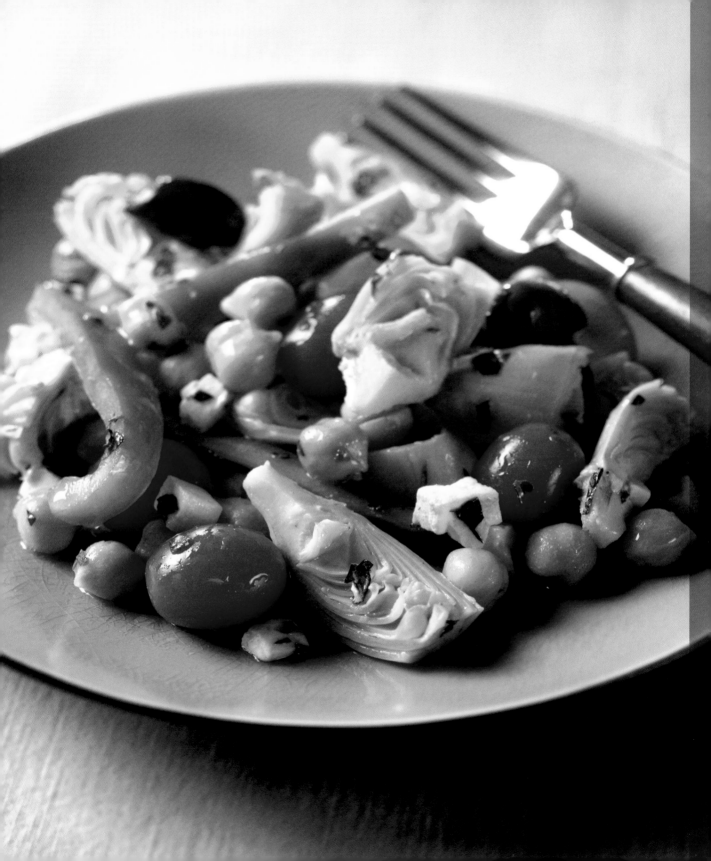

SPICY MEDITERRANEAN WHITE BEAN HUMMUS

YIELD 4 servings | **SERVING SIZE** 2 tablespoons hummus + 4 pita wedges

Although chickpeas are normally used in hummus, white beans offer a refreshing alternative in this unique twist on a classic dish. Adding canola oil to the mixture gives it a silky texture.

1 whole-wheat pita pocket, cut in half crosswise, forming 2 circles

½ of 7.75-ounce can navy beans, rinsed and drained

3 tablespoons plain nonfat yogurt

½ cup (2 ounces) roasted red peppers, drained

2 tablespoons chopped fresh basil leaves

2 medium cloves garlic, peeled

1 tablespoon canola oil

1 teaspoon Louisiana-style hot sauce

⅛ teaspoon salt

Roasted red peppers, chopped, for garnish

1 Preheat oven to 350°F.

2 Cut each pita round into eight wedges. Place them on a baking sheet and bake 4 minutes or until lightly golden. Cool completely on a baking sheet on a wire rack.

3 Meanwhile, put remaining ingredients in blender, secure lid, and purée until smooth.

4 Serve hummus with pita wedges and garnish with chopped roasted peppers.

Calories 125	Cholesterol 0 mg	
Calories from fat 35	Sodium 260 mg	**EXCHANGES PER SERVING**
Total fat 4.0 g	Total carbohydrate 19 g	
Saturated fat 0.3 g	Dietary fiber 3 g	1 starch
Trans fat 0.0 g	Sugars 2 g	1 fat
	Protein 5 g	

Flavorful tip For even more color and flavor punch, sprinkle additional chopped basil on top of the hummus right before serving.

CRUNCHY RED PEPPER-GINGER RELISH
with Cucumber Rounds

YIELD 6 servings | **SERVING SIZE** 6 cucumber slices + 2 tablespoons relish

This appetizer is a great opener—it is light, fresh, and flavorful.

½ cup finely chopped red bell pepper

¼ cup chopped pickled ginger

2 tablespoons finely chopped red onion

1 tablespoon chopped fresh cilantro leaves

1 teaspoon orange zest

1½ tablespoons pourable sugar substitute

2 tablespoons fresh lemon juice

1 tablespoon canola oil

⅛ teaspoon dried red pepper flakes

2 medium cucumbers, cut into ¼-inch-thick slices (18 per cucumber)

1 Combine all ingredients, except cucumbers, in a small bowl. Let stand 30 minutes in the refrigerator, stir, and drain liquids.

2 Serve in another small bowl with a spoon and cucumber slices on the side.

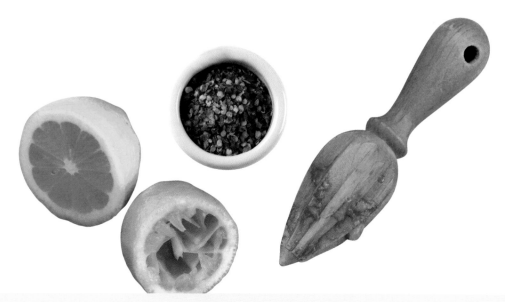

Calories 45	Cholesterol 0 mg	
Calories from fat 20	Sodium 105 mg	**EXCHANGES PER SERVING**
Total fat 2.5 g	Total carbohydrate 5 g	1 vegetable
Saturated fat 0.2 g	Dietary fiber 1 g	½ fat
Trans fat 0.0 g	Sugars 3 g	
	Protein 1 g	

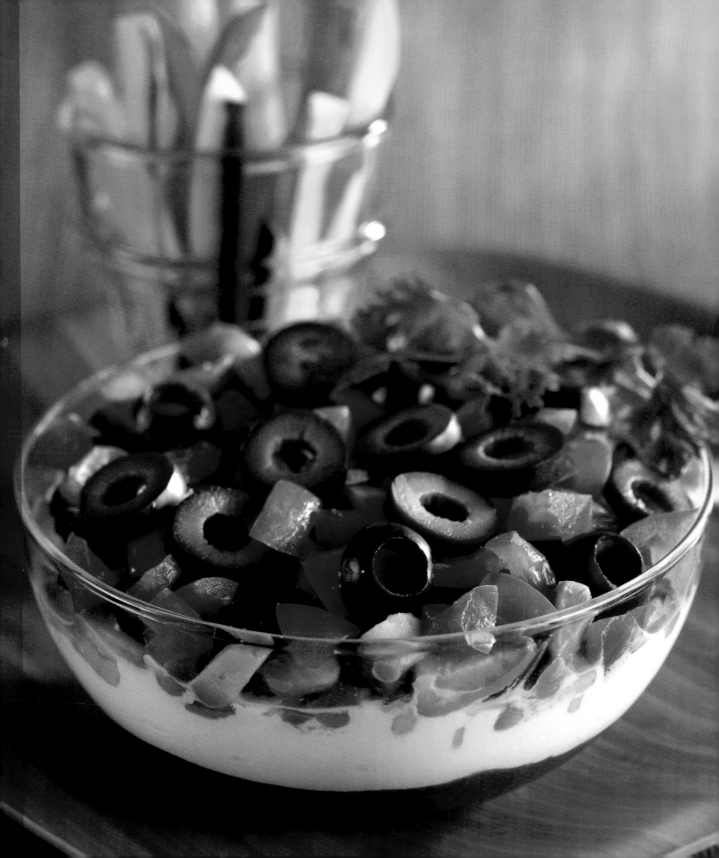

CREAMY BLACK BEAN STACK DIP

YIELD 16 servings | **SERVING SIZE** ⅓ cup

With this no-bake, colorful recipe, you'll never toil over the perfect potluck dish again!

1 can (15 ounces) black beans, rinsed and drained
½ cup mild or medium picante sauce
3 tablespoons fresh lime juice
2 tablespoons canola oil
1 tablespoon chopped fresh cilantro leaves, plus sprig for garnish
1 medium clove garlic, peeled
½ teaspoon ground cumin
1 container (12 ounces) fat-free sour cream
1 ripe medium avocado, peeled, seeded, and diced
1 medium tomato, seeded and diced
1 can (2.25 ounces) sliced ripe olives, drained
1 tablespoon fresh lime juice
Fresh vegetables, sliced for dipping

1 Combine beans, picante sauce, juice, canola oil, cilantro, garlic, and cumin in a blender or small food processor, secure lid, and purée until smooth. Place mixture in a 9-inch pie pan and spread evenly over all using the back of a spoon. Top with remaining ingredients in the order listed.

2 Serve with a variety of fresh vegetables for dipping, such as sliced cucumber, yellow squash, and bell pepper. Garnish dip with sprig of cilantro.

Fresh tip Adding the lime juice at the end prevents the avocados from discoloring.

Calories 80	Cholesterol 0 mg
Calories from fat 35	Sodium 125 mg
Total fat 4.0 g	Total carbohydrate 6 g
Saturated fat 0.4 g	Dietary fiber 2 g
Trans fat 0.0 g	Sugars 1 g
	Protein 3 g

EXCHANGES PER SERVING
½ starch
1 fat

MINI POTATOES WITH CARAMELIZED ONIONS
and Blue Cheese

YIELD 6 servings | **SERVING SIZE** 2 potato halves

The blue cheese in this recipe adds moisture to the potatoes, while the canola oil protects the sugar from burning, giving the onions a rich, deep flavor.

1 tablespoon canola oil

1½ cups very thinly sliced red onions

2 teaspoons sugar

1 teaspoon balsamic vinegar

6 new potatoes (12 ounces total), pierced several times with a fork

⅛ teaspoon salt

¼ cup (1 ounce) blue cheese, crumbled

1 Heat canola oil in a large nonstick skillet over medium-high heat. Add onions and sugar; cook 10 minutes or until richly browned, stirring frequently. Add vinegar; cook 15 seconds. Remove from heat.

2 Meanwhile, microwave potatoes on high 7–8 minutes or until fork-tender. Cut each potato in half lengthwise and place on a serving platter cut side up. Sprinkle evenly with salt and top with blue cheese. Place equal amounts of onion mixture onto potatoes. Cool to room temperature before serving.

		EXCHANGES PER SERVING	
Calories 100	Cholesterol 5 mg		
Calories from fat 35	Sodium 120 mg	1 starch	
Total fat 4.0 g	Total carbohydrate 15 g	½ fat	
Saturated fat 1.0 g	Dietary fiber 1 g		
Trans fat 0.0 g	Sugars 3 g		
	Protein 2 g		

Fast tip It's easier to use a fork when placing the onions on the potatoes.

SOY-MARINATED MUSHROOMS
with Cilantro and Basil

YIELD 4 servings | **SERVING SIZE** about 5 mushrooms

This appetizer is the perfect prelude to an Asian entrée.

- 1 package (8 ounces) medium whole mushrooms, wiped clean with a damp cloth
- ¼ cup finely chopped whole green onions
- 2 tablespoons reduced-sodium soy sauce
- 2 tablespoons fresh lime juice
- 2 tablespoons chopped fresh cilantro leaves
- 2 tablespoons chopped fresh basil leaves
- 1 tablespoon canola oil

1 Combine all ingredients in a gallon-size resealable plastic bag. Seal and shake back and forth several times to coat mushrooms. Refrigerate at least 8 hours or up to 24 hours.

2 To serve, drain mushrooms and discard marinade. Place mushrooms in a small bowl and serve with wooden picks.

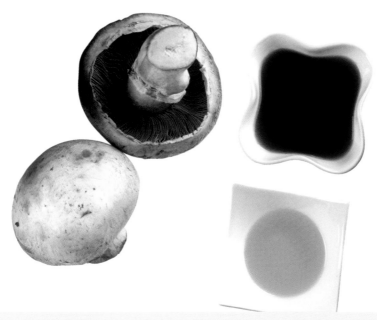

Fresh tip The lime and soy sauce soften the mushrooms while they are marinating and the canola oil helps make the mushrooms tender and plump.

Calories 25
  Calories from fat 15
Total fat 1.5 g
  Saturated fat 0.1 g
  Trans fat 0.0 g

Cholesterol 0 mg
Sodium 100 mg
Total carbohydrate 2 g
  Dietary fiber 1 g
  Sugars 1 g
Protein 2 g

EXCHANGES
PER SERVING
1 vegetable

CRISPY BAKED ZUCCHINI SPEARS
with Lemon

YIELD 6 servings | **SERVING SIZE** 3 spears

Panko are flaky Japanese bread crumbs with a coarser texture than the traditional variety that give a crunchier, lighter crust. Panko and seasonings jazz up zucchini here.

3 small zucchini (12 ounces total), halved and cut into sixths lengthwise
¼ cup fat-free Italian salad dressing
½ cup panko bread crumbs
⅓ cup yellow cornmeal
¾ teaspoon paprika
¼ teaspoon dried thyme leaves
½ teaspoon black pepper
2 tablespoons canola oil
¼ teaspoon salt
2 medium lemons, cut into wedges
Canola oil cooking spray

1 Preheat oven to 450°F.

2 Place zucchini pieces and salad dressing in a medium bowl. Toss gently, yet thoroughly, to coat well.

3 Combine bread crumbs, cornmeal, paprika, thyme, black pepper, and canola oil in a shallow pan, such as a pie pan. Working with five or six zucchini pieces at a time, coat them with bread crumb mixture, pressing lightly with your fingertips to allow the bread crumbs to adhere to zucchini.

4 Coat a large nonstick baking sheet with cooking spray, arrange zucchini pieces in a single layer on the baking sheet, and bake 15 minutes or until golden. Remove from oven and sprinkle evenly with salt.

5 Serve with lemon wedges to squeeze evenly over all.

Calories 105
  Calories from fat 45
Total fat 5.0 g
  Saturated fat 0.4 g
  Trans fat 0.0 g

Cholesterol 0 mg
Sodium 215 mg
Total carbohydrate 14 g
  Dietary fiber 1 g
  Sugars 3 g
Protein 2 g

EXCHANGES PER SERVING
1 starch
1 fat

Flavorful tip Coating the baking sheet with canola oil cooking spray and using canola oil in the zucchini coating helps brown the spears, giving crispy "fried" results in the oven.

MINI CORN CAKES
with Chipotle Aioli

YIELD 4 servings | **SERVING SIZE** 4 corn cakes

Aioli is traditionally a creamy garlic dip. Chipotle aioli serves up smoky, subtle heat while complementing the corn cakes.

AIOLI

- ⅓ cup fat-free sour cream
- ½–¾ teaspoon adobo sauce
- 2–3 tablespoons fat-free milk or water
- ½ medium clove garlic, minced
- ⅛ teaspoon salt

CORN CAKES

- 2 large egg whites
- 1 tablespoon canola mayonnaise
- 1½ cups frozen corn kernels, thawed and patted dry
- ½ cup finely chopped red bell pepper
- ¼ cup finely chopped green onions
- 2 tablespoons chopped fresh parsley leaves
- ¼ cup cornmeal
- ¼ teaspoon salt
- ¼ teaspoon black pepper
- Canola oil cooking spray
- 1 tablespoon canola oil, divided

1 Combine sour cream and adobo sauce in a small bowl, add remaining aioli ingredients, and stir until smooth. Set aside.

2 Combine egg whites and canola mayonnaise in a medium bowl and stir until well blended. Stir in remaining corn cake ingredients, except cooking spray and canola oil.

3 Coat a large nonstick skillet with cooking spray, add ½ tablespoon canola oil to skillet, and heat over medium heat. Tilt skillet to lightly coat bottom of pan. Working in two batches, spoon rounded tablespoon of corn mixture into skillet, making eight mounds. Flatten slightly for an even thickness, cook 2 minutes on each side or until golden, and place on a serving platter. Repeat with remaining canola oil and corn mixture.

4 Serve corn cakes with aioli.

Fast tip Adobo sauce can be purchased in a jar or taken from canned chipotle chile peppers packed in the sauce.

Calories 150
Calories from fat 45
Total fat 5.0 g
Saturated fat 0.3 g
Trans fat 0.0 g

Cholesterol 0 mg
Sodium 295 mg
Total carbohydrate 20 g
Dietary fiber 2 g
Sugars 4 g
Protein 6 g

EXCHANGES PER SERVING
1 starch
1 vegetable
1 fat

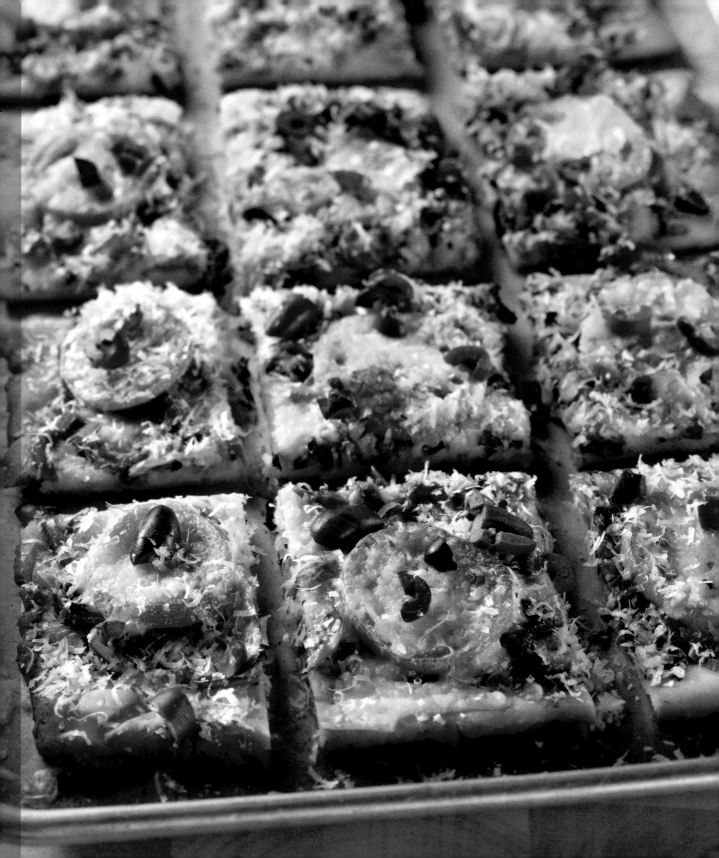

BASIL FOCACCIA WEDGES

YIELD 12 servings | **SERVING SIZE** 2 pieces

These healthy mini pizzas will inspire children to eat vegetables! The canola oil browns the vegetables, brings out their rich flavors, and gives the dough a crispy crust.

1½ tablespoons canola oil, divided

1 cup thinly sliced green bell pepper

½ cup thinly sliced red onion

½ package (8 ounces) sliced mushrooms

2 medium cloves garlic, minced

1 package (13.8 ounces) focaccia-style, refrigerated pizza dough

¼ teaspoon dried red pepper flakes

½ cup chopped fresh basil leaves

2 small plum tomatoes, cut into 12 rounds total

½ cup (2 ounces) shredded part-skim mozzarella

2 tablespoons grated Parmesan cheese

16 pitted kalamata olives, chopped

1 Preheat oven to 400°F. Heat 1 tablespoon canola oil in a large nonstick skillet over medium-high heat. Add bell pepper and onions; cook 2 minutes. Add mushrooms; cook 2 minutes, using two utensils to stir easily. Add garlic, cook 15 seconds, and set aside.

2 Drizzle remaining ½ tablespoon canola oil on a baking sheet. Use fingertips to spread oil evenly. Unroll dough onto baking sheet and shape into an 11 × 8-inch rectangle. Top dough with pepper flakes and mushroom mixture, spooning as close to edges as possible. Top with basil and arrange tomatoes in 12 even sections.

3 Bake 12 minutes. Sprinkle evenly with mozzarella. Bake 6 more minutes or until deep golden on edges. Top with Parmesan and sprinkle evenly with olives. Allow to cool to room temperature.

4 When serving, cut into 12 squares, and then cut each square in half diagonally to make 24 pieces total.

Fast tip Using the prongs of a fork helps distribute the vegetables evenly on top of the uncooked dough. A pizza cutter allows for easier slicing of the wedges.

Calories 125	Cholesterol 5 mg
Calories from fat 40	Sodium 320 mg
Total fat 4.5 g	Total carbohydrate 18 g
Saturated fat 1.1 g	Dietary fiber 1 g
Trans fat 0.0 g	Sugars 3 g
	Protein 5 g

EXCHANGES PER SERVING

1 starch
1 fat

MINI VEGETABLE PANINI

YIELD 4 servings | **SERVING SIZE** 2 panini

Get a taste of Italy with this fun, easy-to-make appetizer. Buon appetito!

6 pitted kalamata olives, finely chopped

1 medium clove garlic, minced

1 tablespoon red wine vinegar

1½ tablespoons canola oil, divided

⅛ teaspoon dried red pepper flakes

½ of 8-ounce whole-wheat baguette, cut into 16 slices

1 medium plum tomato, cut into 8 slices

12 medium basil leaves

1 slice (¾ ounce) reduced-fat provolone or Swiss cheese, cut into 8 wedges

1 Combine olives, garlic, vinegar, ½ tablespoon canola oil, and pepper flakes in a small bowl and stir until well blended.

2 Place 8 bread slices on a clean work surface. Top each with about 1 teaspoon olive mixture, tomato slice, basil leaf, cheese wedge, and another bread slice. Press down firmly to allow ingredients to adhere slightly.

3 Heat remaining 1 tablespoon canola oil in a large nonstick skillet over medium heat. Add sandwiches and top with a dinner plate and 3–4 bread plates or cans of vegetables to weigh down sandwiches as they cook. Cook 3 minutes, turn, and cook 2–3 minutes or until golden on bottom and cheese has melted.

Calories 150
　Calories from fat 70
Total fat 8.0 g
　Saturated fat 1.5 g
　Trans fat 0.0 g

Cholesterol 5 mg
Sodium 225 mg
Total carbohydrate 14 g
　Dietary fiber 3 g
　Sugars 2 g
Protein 6 g

EXCHANGES
PER SERVING
1 starch
1½ fat

WEST INDIES SHRIMP AND JALAPEÑO ROUNDS

YIELD 4 servings | **SERVING SIZE** about 4 shrimp

This appetizer offers flavors characteristic of the tropics without too much heat. The canola oil in the marinade calms down the heat from the jalapeño, so it doesn't overpower the other ingredients.

¼ cup water

1 teaspoon seafood seasoning

½ lb medium raw shrimp, peeled and deveined

1 medium jalapeño, stemmed and thinly sliced into rounds

¼ cup thinly sliced red onion

2 tablespoons chopped fresh parsley leaves

1 tablespoon capers, drained

1 teaspoon dried oregano leaves, crushed

2 tablespoons white wine vinegar

1 tablespoon canola oil

1 medium clove garlic, minced

1 Bring water and seafood seasoning to a boil in a medium saucepan over high heat. Add shrimp and return to boil. Reduce heat and simmer, uncovered, 3–4 minutes or until opaque in center. Drain well. Place shrimp in a shallow pan, such as a pie pan, and refrigerate until completely cooled.

2 Combine remaining ingredients in a medium bowl.

3 To serve, combine shrimp with jalapeño mixture. Let stand 15 minutes, stirring frequently. Serve with wooden picks.

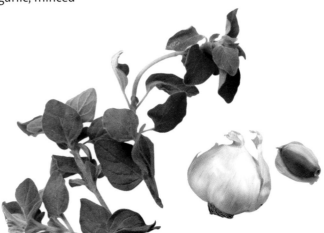

Fast tip The shrimp and marinade can be prepared separately in advance and stored in the refrigerator until ready to serve. For peak flavors, serve after 15 minutes of marinating.

Calories 85
Calories from fat 35
Total fat 4.0 g
Saturated fat 0.4 g
Trans fat 0.0 g

Cholesterol 80 mg
Sodium 240 mg
Total carbohydrate 2 g
Dietary fiber 1 g
Sugars 1 g
Protein 9 g

EXCHANGES PER SERVING
1 lean meat
½ fat

PORK SLIDERS
with Raspberry Mustard Sauce

YIELD 12 servings | **SERVING SIZE** 2 sliders

These sandwiches are great for a tailgate party. They will "slide" right into the mouths of sports fans! The sauce gets its game on thanks to the sharp mustard, sweet fruit spread, and creamy canola mayonnaise.

SLIDERS

- ½ teaspoon garlic powder
- ½ teaspoon dried thyme leaves
- ½ teaspoon coarsely ground black pepper
- 1 lb pork tenderloin
- 1 tablespoon canola oil
  Canola oil cooking spray
- 12 wheat or multigrain mini rolls, halved

SAUCE

- ¼ cup raspberry fruit spread
- 2 tablespoons coarse-grain Dijon mustard
- 2 tablespoons canola mayonnaise
- 1 teaspoon pourable sugar substitute
- ¼ teaspoon ground allspice
- ⅛ teaspoon dried red pepper flakes (optional)

1 Preheat oven to 425°F. Combine garlic powder, thyme, and black pepper in a small bowl. Sprinkle both sides of pork tenderloin with garlic powder mixture. Heat canola oil in a large nonstick skillet over medium-high heat. Add pork, cook 3 minutes, turn, and cook 2 more minutes or until richly browned. Remove from heat.

2 Coat a foil-lined baking sheet with cooking spray, place pork on baking sheet, and cook 18–20 minutes, until barely pink in center. Place on a cutting board and let stand 5 minutes before thinly slicing. If desired, wrap rolls in foil and place in oven 5 minutes to warm before serving.

3 Place fruit spread in a microwave-safe small bowl. Cover and microwave on high for 20 seconds or until slightly melted. Stir in remaining sauce ingredients until well blended.

4 To serve, place pork on a serving platter and sauce in another small bowl. Serve with rolls.

Calories 140
  Calories from fat 35
Total fat 4.0 g
  Saturated fat 0.6 g
  Trans fat 0.0 g

Cholesterol 20 mg
Sodium 210 mg
Total carbohydrate 17 g
  Dietary fiber 2 g
  Sugars 5 g
Protein 10 g

EXCHANGES PER SERVING
1 starch
1 lean meat
½ fat

Fresh tip For a change of pace, you can substitute apricot fruit spread for raspberry.

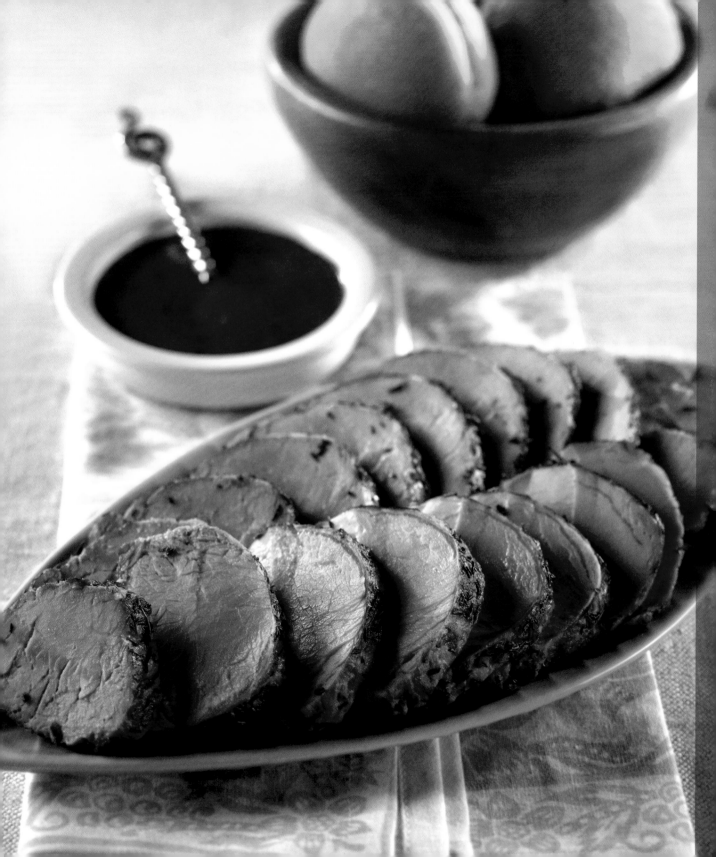

MINI GREEK CHICKEN KABOBS

YIELD 8 servings | **SERVING SIZE** 2 kabobs

No matter what time of year it is, you will think of summer when grilling these colorful kabobs.

MARINADE

1½ tablespoons canola oil

½ teaspoon lemon zest

1–2 tablespoons fresh lemon juice

1½ teaspoons Worcestershire sauce

1½ teaspoons dried oregano leaves

½ teaspoon dried dill

1 medium clove garlic, minced

⅛ teaspoon dried red pepper flakes

¼ teaspoon salt

KABOBS

Canola oil cooking spray

4 chicken tenders (8 ounces total), rinsed and patted dry, each cut into fourths crosswise

½ small green bell pepper, cut into 16 cubes

16 grape tomatoes

1 small yellow squash, quartered lengthwise and cut into 16 pieces

16 bamboo skewers (6 inches each)

1 Combine marinade ingredients in a quart-sized resealable plastic bag, seal tightly, and toss back and forth until well blended. Remove 2 tablespoons mixture, place in a small bowl, and set aside. Add chicken pieces to bag with remaining marinade, seal tightly, and toss back and forth to coat completely. Refrigerate 1 hour, turning occasionally.

2 Coat grill rack with cooking spray and preheat grill to medium-high heat.

3 Remove chicken from marinade and discard marinade. Thread piece of chicken and each vegetable per skewer in this order: pepper, chicken, tomato, and squash. Repeat with remaining skewers.

4 Place skewers on a grill rack and cook 5 minutes or until chicken is no longer pink in the center and juices run clear, turning frequently and being careful not to overcook. Remove from grill, place on a serving platter, and brush reserved 2 tablespoons marinade evenly over all. Serve warm.

Calories 60
    Calories from fat 25
Total fat 3.0 g
    Saturated fat 0.4 g
    Trans fat 0.0 g

Cholesterol 15 mg
Sodium 80 mg
Total carbohydrate 2 g
    Dietary fiber 1 g
    Sugars 1 g
Protein 6 g

EXCHANGES PER SERVING
1 lean meat
½ fat

Flavorful tip Turn contents during the marinating time to ensure even coating.

APRICOT HOISIN-GLAZED MEATBALLS

YIELD 4 servings | **SERVING SIZE** 6 meatballs

Meatballs are a popular appetizer at any gathering, and these are healthier than the average ones. The glaze tastes more complex than just three ingredients because of the use of highly seasoned hoisin sauce.

MEATBALLS

- 1 lb 96% extra-lean ground beef
- 2 medium whole green onions, trimmed and finely chopped
- ¼ cup quick-cooking oats
- 2 egg whites
- 1 tablespoon grated fresh ginger
- 1 tablespoon canola oil

GLAZE

- 3 tablespoons hoisin sauce
- 2 tablespoons water
- ⅔ cup apricot fruit spread

1 Combine meatball ingredients, except canola oil, in a medium bowl and shape into 24 meatballs.

2 Heat canola oil in a large nonstick skillet over medium-high heat. Add meatballs and cook 10 minutes or until juices run clear and no pink is inside, turning frequently. Stir using a fork and heat-resistant rubber spatula to turn easily and gently. Remove from heat; set aside on a separate plate.

3 To pan residue, add glaze ingredients and cook 1 minute, stirring frequently. Add meatballs and cook 3 minutes or until glazed and reduced slightly, stirring frequently. Remove from heat and let stand 5 minutes to thicken slightly, stirring occasionally.

4 Serve with wooden picks.

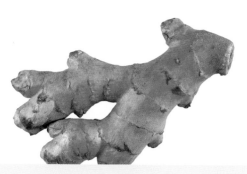

Fresh tip The meatballs may be served as an entrée over 2 cups of cooked brown rice and tossed with chopped green onions.

Calories 330
  Calories from fat 80
Total fat 9.0 g
  Saturated fat 2.4 g
  Trans fat 0.3 g

Cholesterol 60 mg
Sodium 280 mg
Total carbohydrate 35 g
  Dietary fiber 1 g
  Sugars 25 g
Protein 27 g

EXCHANGES PER SERVING
2½ carbohydrate
4 lean meat

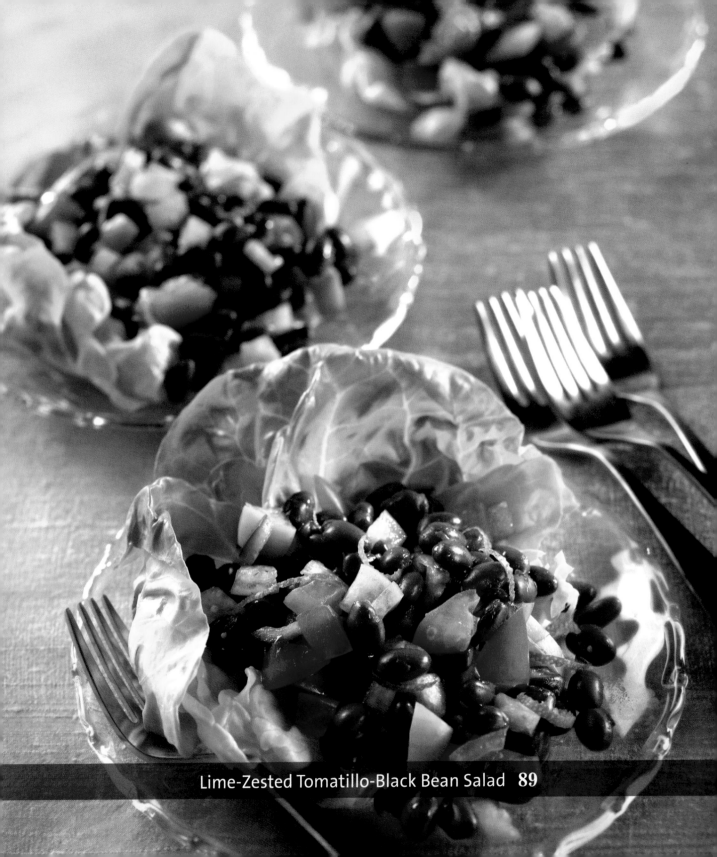

Lime-Zested Tomatillo-Black Bean Salad **89**

SALADS

White Bean and Roasted Red Pepper Salad | 88

Lime-Zested Tomatillo-Black Bean Salad | 89

Sweet Grape Tomato and Poblano Salad | 90

Greek Garbanzo Salsa Salad | 91

Jicama and Sweet Lemon Salad | 93

Fresh Broccoli and Dried Cranberry Salad | 94

Asian Vegetable Slaw | 95

Sweet Pineapple-Ginger Slaw | 96

Baby Spinach and Prosciutto with Sherry Vinaigrette | 97

Roasted Beet and Carrot Salad | 98

Mixed Greens, String Beans, and Walnuts with White Wine-Raspberry Vinaigrette | 100

Simple Fresh Herb Salad | 101

Sweet and Crispy Cucumber-Anaheim Salad | 102

Barley-Artichoke Salad on Romaine | 103

Quinoa and Browned Onion Salad with Apples | 105

Asparagus-Wheat Berry Salad with Blue Cheese | 106

Wilted Kale Salad | 107

Spinach Salad with Grilled and Fresh Fruit | 108

WHITE BEAN AND ROASTED RED PEPPER SALAD

YIELD 12 servings | **SERVING SIZE** 1/3 cup bean mixture + 3/4 cup spinach

The coarsely chopped spinach in this dish not only provides great color, but also packs more vitamins and minerals into every serving.

- 1/2 of 15-ounce can no-salt-added navy beans, rinsed and drained
- 1 cup grape tomatoes, quartered
- 1 cup (1/2 ounce) loosely packed baby spinach, coarsely chopped
- 1/2 cup chopped roasted red peppers
- 8 pitted kalamata olives, coarsely chopped
- 2 tablespoons chopped fresh basil leaves
- 1 medium clove garlic, minced
- 1 tablespoon canola oil
- 1 tablespoon cider vinegar
- 3 cups (1 1/2 ounces) loosely packed baby spinach leaves

1 Combine beans, tomatoes, chopped spinach, peppers, olives, basil, and garlic in a medium bowl.

2 To serve, add canola oil and vinegar. Using a rubber spatula, toss ingredients gently, yet thoroughly, until well coated. Place equal amounts of whole spinach leaves on four salad plates and spoon bean mixture on top.

		EXCHANGES PER SERVING
Calories 105	Cholesterol 0 mg	
Calories from fat 40	Sodium 115 mg	1/2 starch
Total fat 4.5 g	Total carbohydrate 12 g	1 vegetable
Saturated fat 0.4 g	Dietary fiber 4 g	1 fat
Trans fat 0.0 g	Sugars 2 g	
	Protein 4 g	

Fast tip The bean mixture may be assembled without the canola oil and vinegar up to 8 hours in advance. Simply cover and refrigerate, then add the canola oil and vinegar at serving time for peak flavors and texture.

LIME-ZESTED TOMATILLO-BLACK BEAN SALAD

YIELD 6 servings | **SERVING SIZE** ½ cup

Tomatillos give a bite to this Latin-inspired dish, so the lime juice and zest are only needed as accents.

- 2 medium tomatillos, papery skin removed and finely chopped
- ½ medium poblano chili pepper, seeded and finely chopped
- 2 medium plum tomatoes, finely chopped
- ½ of 15-ounce can black beans, rinsed and drained
- 2–3 tablespoons chopped fresh cilantro leaves (optional)
- 1 teaspoon lime zest
- 1 ripe medium avocado, peeled, pitted, and diced
- 1 tablespoon fresh lime juice
- 1 tablespoon canola oil
- ¼ teaspoon salt
- 6 Boston Bibb lettuce leaves or medium romaine leaves

1 Combine tomatillos, poblano pepper, tomatoes, beans, cilantro, and zest in a medium bowl.

2 When ready to serve, add remaining ingredients and stir gently, yet thoroughly, until well blended. Serve on lettuce leaves.

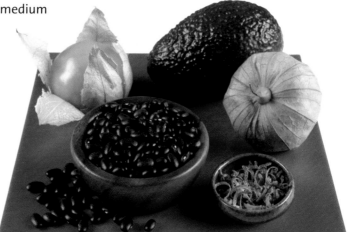

Fresh tip This salad may be served as an appetizer on cucumber rounds.

Calories 100	Cholesterol 0 mg	
Calories from fat 55	Sodium 130 mg	**EXCHANGES PER SERVING**
Total fat 6.0 g	Total carbohydrate 9 g	½ starch
Saturated fat 0.8 g	Dietary fiber 4 g	1 fat
Trans fat 0.0 g	Sugars 2 g	
	Protein 3 g	

SWEET GRAPE TOMATO AND POBLANO SALAD

YIELD 4 servings | **SERVING SIZE** ³/₄ cup

Grape tomatoes have a concentrated and sweet flavor. They give the taste of "in season" all year long. Poblano pepper with the tomatoes adds another layer of flavor.

1 pint grape tomatoes, halved
1 medium poblano, seeded, thinly sliced, and cut into 2-inch strips (or 1 small green bell pepper and ¹/₈ teaspoon dried red pepper flakes)
¹/₄ cup finely chopped red onion
2 tablespoons chopped fresh cilantro leaves
2 tablespoons fresh lime juice
2 tablespoons cider vinegar
1 tablespoon canola oil
1 medium clove garlic, minced
¹/₄ teaspoon salt

1 Combine all ingredients in a medium bowl and toss gently, yet thoroughly, until well blended. Let stand 10 minutes before serving.

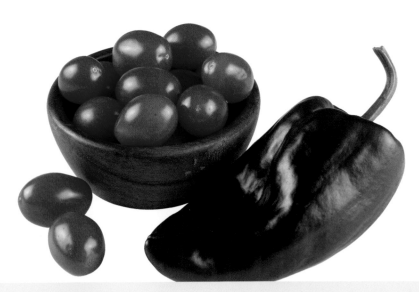

Calories 60
 Calories from fat 30
Total fat 3.5 g
 Saturated fat 0.3 g
 Trans fat 0.0 g
Cholesterol 0 mg
Sodium 150 mg
Total carbohydrate 7 g
 Dietary fiber 1 g
 Sugars 4 g
Protein 1 g

EXCHANGES PER SERVING
1 vegetable
1 fat

Flavorful tip Allowing the salad to stand 10 minutes helps blend the flavors without the ingredients losing their pronounced flavors. For peak flavors and texture, however, serve within 30 minutes.

GREEK GARBANZO SALSA SALAD

YIELD 4 servings | **SERVING SIZE** ¾ cup

This recipe proves that salsa shouldn't be limited to traditional ingredients. Chickpeas, also known as garbanzo beans, are a good vegetarian source of protein.

5	medium sun-dried tomato halves
½	cup boiling water
½	of 16-ounce can chickpeas, rinsed and drained
½	of 13.75-ounce can quartered artichoke hearts, drained and coarsely chopped
¼	of 8-ounce package whole mushrooms, cleaned and chopped
½	cup chopped roasted red peppers
8–12	pepperoncini peppers, chopped (about 2–3 ounces total)
1½	tablespoons canola oil
¼	cup (1 ounce) crumbled reduced-fat feta cheese
1	teaspoon dried oregano leaves
1	medium clove garlic, minced
4	cups loosely packed baby spinach

1 Place sun-dried tomatoes in a small bowl, add boiling water, and let stand 2 minutes to soften slightly. Drain and place on a cutting board to cool slightly, about 2 minutes, before chopping.

2 Meanwhile, combine remaining ingredients, except spinach, in a medium bowl. Add chopped tomatoes to artichoke mixture. Toss gently, yet thoroughly, until well blended. Let stand 15 minutes before serving. Serve on baby spinach divided equally on four plates.

Fresh tip Chop the ingredients smaller or into chunkier pieces for a refreshing new twist on the salsa or salad. A medium cucumber, peeled and sliced, may be substituted for the baby spinach.

Calories 155	Cholesterol 0 mg	**EXCHANGES PER SERVING**
Calories from fat 65	Sodium 380 mg	½ starch
Total fat 7.0 g	Total carbohydrate 16 g	1 vegetable
Saturated fat 1.2 g	Dietary fiber 5 g	1 lean meat
Trans fat 0.0 g	Sugars 5 g	1 fat
	Protein 7 g	

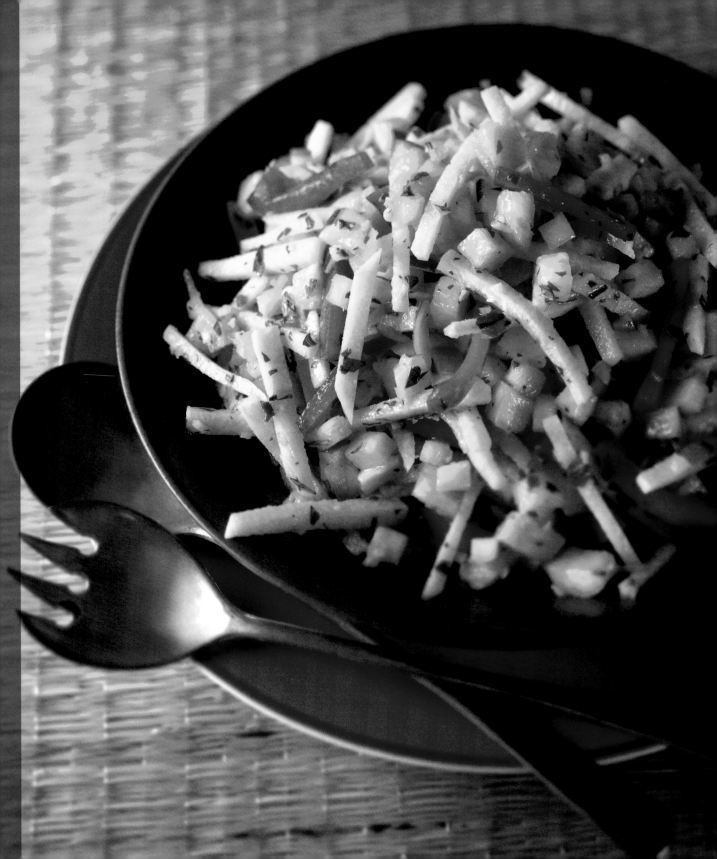

JICAMA AND SWEET LEMON SALAD

YIELD 8 servings | **SERVING SIZE** 1/2 cup

This crisp and refreshing salad is ideal for dining outdoors in the summer sun.

1 small jicama (about 8 ounces total), peeled, thinly sliced, and cut into matchstick-size pieces (about 1½ cups total)

½ medium red bell pepper, thinly sliced and cut into 2-inch-long pieces

1 cup diced fresh pineapple

2 tablespoons chopped fresh cilantro leaves

¼ cup finely chopped red onion

1 teaspoon lemon zest

3 tablespoons fresh lemon juice

2 tablespoons pourable sugar substitute

2 tablespoons canola oil

2 teaspoons grated fresh ginger

⅛ teaspoon dried red pepper flakes

1 Combine all ingredients in a large bowl and toss gently, yet thoroughly, until well blended. Let stand 15 minutes before serving.

Fresh tip Jicama, also known as Mexican turnip, has crispy white flesh like a raw potato and the subtle taste of a pear. Jicama can be found in major supermarkets, but if it is not available, you can substitute firm pears.

Calories 60
  Calories from fat 30
Total fat 3.5 g
  Saturated fat 0.3 g
  Trans fat 0.0 g

Cholesterol 0 mg
Sodium 0 mg
Total carbohydrate 7 g
  Dietary fiber 2 g
  Sugars 3 g
Protein 0 g

EXCHANGES PER SERVING
1 vegetable
½ fat

FRESH BROCCOLI AND DRIED CRANBERRY SALAD

YIELD 4 servings | **SERVING SIZE** ¾ cup

Everyone loves broccoli salad and this one with dried cranberries is sure to please with its blend of sweet and savory flavors.

2 tablespoons sunflower seeds
½ cup water
2 cups small broccoli florets
½ cup matchstick carrots
½ cup dried cranberries
¼ cup finely chopped red onion
1 tablespoon canola oil
2 teaspoons cider vinegar
⅛ teaspoon salt
⅛ teaspoon dried red pepper flakes

1 Heat a medium nonstick skillet over medium-high heat. Add sunflower seeds; cook 2 minutes or until beginning to brown lightly, stirring frequently. Remove from skillet and set aside on a separate plate.

2 Add water to skillet and bring to a boil over medium-high heat. Add broccoli, cover tightly, and cook 1 minute. Immediately drain broccoli in a colander, run under cold water to cool quickly, shake off excess liquid, and pat dry with paper towels.

3 Place broccoli in a medium bowl with remaining ingredients. Toss to combine.

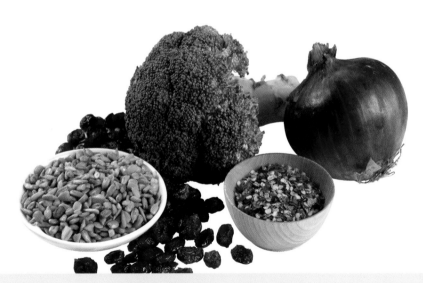

		EXCHANGES PER SERVING	
Calories 120	Cholesterol 0 mg	1 fruit	*Fresh tip* Cooking the broccoli briefly,
Calories from fat 55	Sodium 90 mg	1 vegetable	then immediately running it under cold
Total fat 6.0 g	Total carbohydrate 18 g	1 fat	water, makes the salad crunchier and
Saturated fat 0.5 g	Dietary fiber 3 g		have a milder broccoli taste.
Trans fat 0.0 g	Sugars 12 g		
	Protein 2 g		

ASIAN VEGETABLE SLAW

Purple-hued cabbage, brilliant green snow peas, and fire-engine red peppers make this slaw jump with eye appeal.

SALAD

- 2 cups loosely packed shredded red cabbage
- ¾ cup fresh (or thawed frozen) snow peas, cut diagonally into 1-inch pieces
- ½ cup frozen shelled edamame, thawed
- ½ cup diced red onion
- ½ medium red bell pepper, cut into thin strips, then into 2-inch pieces
- ⅓ cup (1½ ounces) slivered almonds, toasted

VINAIGRETTE

- 2 tablespoons reduced-sodium soy sauce
- 2 tablespoons cider vinegar
- 2 tablespoons pourable sugar substitute
- 1 tablespoon canola oil
- ⅛ teaspoon dried red pepper flakes (optional)

1 Combine salad ingredients in a medium bowl. Combine vinaigrette ingredients in a small jar, secure lid, and shake vigorously until well blended.

2 At time of serving, pour vinaigrette over salad ingredients and toss gently, yet thoroughly, to coat completely.

Fresh tip Double or triple the vinaigrette and store it in the refrigerator to have on hand for breaks from traditional vinaigrettes. Try the vinaigrette on spring greens, red onion, and fruits, such as mandarin oranges or strawberries.

Calories 105	Cholesterol 0 mg
Calories from fat 65	Sodium 195 mg
Total fat 7.0 g	Total carbohydrate 8 g
Saturated fat 0.6 g	Dietary fiber 3 g
Trans fat 0.0 g	Sugars 4 g
	Protein 4 g

EXCHANGES PER SERVING
1 vegetable
1½ fat

SWEET PINEAPPLE-GINGER SLAW

YIELD 6 servings | **SERVING SIZE** ⅔ cup

Pickled ginger, pineapple, and mint make this unique coleslaw zesty.

4 cups finely shredded cabbage

2 medium whole green onions, diagonally sliced

1 can (8 ounces) pineapple tidbits in own juice, drained

½ cup chopped fresh mint leaves

¼ cup chopped pickled ginger

3 tablespoons fresh lime juice

2 tablespoons pourable sugar substitute

1 tablespoon canola oil

1 Combine all ingredients in a large bowl. Using two utensils, toss gently, yet thoroughly, until well blended. Cover with plastic wrap and refrigerate 30 minutes before serving.

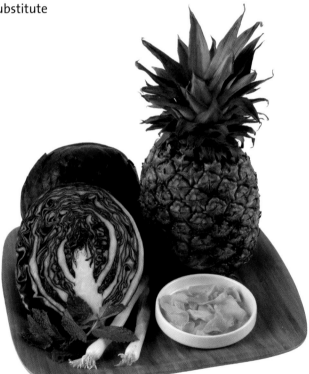

Calories 55
    Calories from fat 20
Total fat 2.5 g
    Saturated fat 0.2 g
    Trans fat 0.0 g

Cholesterol 0 mg
Sodium 110 mg
Total carbohydrate 8 g
    Dietary fiber 2 g
    Sugars 6 g
Protein 1 g

EXCHANGES PER SERVING
½ carbohydrate
½ fat

Flavorful tip Chop thin strips of the pickled ginger for peak flavors and texture. This ingredient is sold in the Asian section of major supermarkets. If you can't find it, use grated fresh ginger instead.

BABY SPINACH AND PROSCIUTTO
with Sherry Vinaigrette

YIELD 4 servings | SERVING SIZE 1½ cups

Add interest and variety to your salads by using high-flavored ingredients, such as sherry and prosciutto.

VINAIGRETTE

- ½ cup dry sherry
- ¼ cup balsamic vinegar
- 3 tablespoons pourable sugar substitute
- 2 tablespoons canola oil
- 4 medium cloves garlic, minced

SALAD

- 1 package (6 ounces) fresh baby spinach
- ½ of 8-ounce package sliced mushrooms
- ½ cup thinly sliced red onion
- 4 thin slices prosciutto (2 ounces), torn or cut into bite-size pieces

1 Combine vinaigrette ingredients in a small jar, secure lid, and shake vigorously until completely blended.

2 Combine spinach, mushrooms, and red onion in a salad bowl. Add ½ cup vinaigrette and toss gently, yet thoroughly, to coat. Top with prosciutto and toss gently again. Refrigerate remaining vinaigrette for later use.

Flavorful tip For variation, cook prosciutto slices in a large nonstick skillet over medium-high heat for 5 minutes or until crisp and then finely chop. Adding flavorful ingredients, such as sherry, to vinaigrette helps stretch it without adding fat.

Calories 105	Cholesterol 10 mg	
Calories from fat 45	Sodium 285 mg	**EXCHANGES**
Total fat 5.0 g	Total carbohydrate 7 g	**PER SERVING**
Saturated fat 0.8 g	Dietary fiber 1 g	1 vegetable
Trans fat 0.0 g	Sugars 3 g	1 medium-fat meat
	Protein 6 g	

ROASTED BEET AND CARROT SALAD

YIELD 4 servings | **SERVING SIZE** 1½ cups

You just can't "beet" the pretty colors in this nutrient-dense salad.

Canola oil cooking spray

SALAD

2 medium beets (about 8 ounces total), peeled, cut into 8 wedges each

1 medium carrot (about 3 ounces), peeled, cut in half lengthwise, and cut into 2-inch pieces

1 medium parsnip (about 3 ounces), peeled, quartered lengthwise, and cut into 2-inch pieces

1 teaspoon canola oil

4 cups (about 4 ounces) packed spring greens

½ cup thinly sliced red onion

¼ cup golden raisins (optional)

¼ cup (1 ounce) pecan pieces, toasted

VINAIGRETTE

3 tablespoons balsamic vinegar

1 tablespoon plus 2 teaspoons canola oil

⅛ teaspoon dried red pepper flakes

1 medium clove garlic, minced

¼ teaspoon salt

¼ teaspoon coarsely ground black pepper

1 Preheat oven to 425°F.

2 Coat a foil-lined baking sheet with cooking spray. Place beets, carrots, and parsnips on baking sheet. Drizzle evenly with 1 teaspoon canola oil and toss gently, yet thoroughly, to coat lightly. Arrange vegetables in a single layer and bake 10 minutes; stir and bake an additional 7 minutes or until beets are just tender when pierced with a fork. Remove from heat and let stand to cool slightly, about 10 minutes.

3 Combine vinaigrette ingredients in a small jar, secure lid, and shake well to blend thoroughly.

4 Arrange equal amounts of salad greens on four salad plates. In the following order, top with equal amounts of onion, roasted vegetables, raisins, and pecans. Spoon vinaigrette evenly over all. Serve immediately for peak flavors.

		EXCHANGES PER SERVING	
Calories 165	Cholesterol 0 mg		
Calories from fat 110	Sodium 185 mg	½ starch	
Total fat 12.0 g	Total carbohydrate 14 g	1 vegetable	
Saturated fat 1.0 g	Dietary fiber 3 g	2 fat	
Trans fat 0.0 g	Sugars 6 g		
	Protein 2 g		

Fast tip To avoid stains when peeling beets, peel them under running water. This rinses the juice away before it has time to come in contact with your fingers.

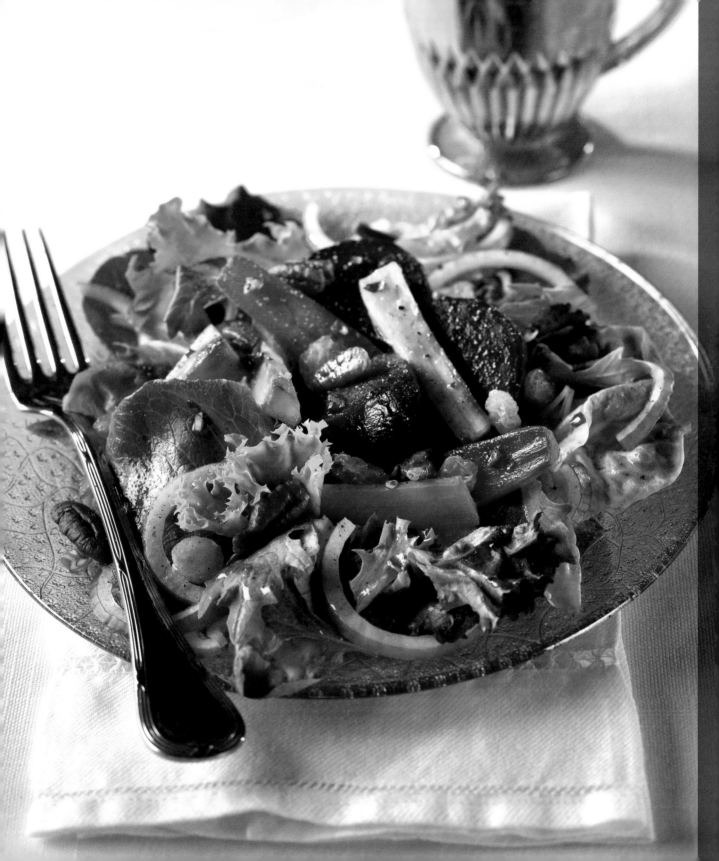

MIXED GREENS, STRING BEANS, AND WALNUTS
with White Wine-Raspberry Vinaigrette

YIELD 4 servings | **SERVING SIZE** 1½ cups

This recipe offers simple elegance by combining wholesome ingredients with a fresh vinaigrette.

SALAD

- ¼ cup (1 ounce) walnut pieces
- 2 cups water
- 1 cup fresh whole green beans, trimmed
- 6 cups (about 6 ounces) loosely packed torn romaine lettuce

VINAIGRETTE

- ½ cup white wine, such as pinot grigio
- ¼ cup raspberry vinegar
- 3 tablespoons coarse-grain Dijon mustard
- 2 tablespoons canola oil
- 2 tablespoons chopped fresh oregano leaves or 2 teaspoons dried oregano leaves
- 1 tablespoon plus 1 teaspoon pourable sugar substitute
- 2 medium cloves garlic, minced
- ½ teaspoon salt
- ½ teaspoon coarsely ground black pepper

1 Place a large saucepan over medium-high heat until hot. Add walnuts and cook 2–3 minutes or until lightly browned, stirring frequently. Remove from saucepan and set aside.

2 Add 2 cups water to saucepan and bring to a boil over high heat. Add beans and return to a boil. Reduce heat and simmer, covered tightly, 4 minutes or until just tender crisp. Immediately drain in a colander and run under cold water to cool quickly. Shake off excess liquid and drain on paper towels.

3 Place romaine in a large salad bowl and top with beans and nuts.

4 Combine vinaigrette ingredients in a jar, secure lid, and shake vigorously until well blended. Pour ½ cup vinaigrette evenly over lettuce mixture and toss gently, yet thoroughly, until well coated. Refrigerate remaining vinaigrette for later use.

Calories 130
  Calories from fat 80
Total fat 9.0 g
  Saturated fat 0.7 g
  Trans fat 0.0 g

Cholesterol 0 mg
Sodium 285 mg
Total carbohydrate 10 g
  Dietary fiber 2 g
  Sugars 5 g
Protein 2 g

EXCHANGES PER SERVING
½ carbohydrate
2 fat

Fresh tip Asparagus will work in place of the green beans, but only cook the asparagus for 1–2 minutes or until just tender crisp.

SIMPLE FRESH HERB SALAD

YIELD 4 servings | **SERVING SIZE** 1½ cups

The fresh basil, oregano, and rosemary have leading roles in this salad. The tomatoes and hearts of palm provide visual effects.

1 package (5 ounces) spring greens
1 tablespoon chopped fresh basil leaves
1 tablespoon chopped fresh oregano leaves
½ teaspoon chopped fresh rosemary leaves
2 tablespoons white balsamic vinegar
1½ tablespoons canola oil
1 teaspoon lemon zest
¼ teaspoon coarsely ground black pepper
¼ teaspoon salt
1 medium tomato, seeded and diced
1 can (14.75 ounces) hearts of palm, drained and cut into ½-inch rounds

1 Place greens in a large salad bowl and sprinkle basil, oregano, and rosemary evenly over all.

2 Combine vinegar, canola oil, zest, pepper, and salt in a small jar. Shake vigorously to mix well. Pour over greens and toss gently, yet thoroughly, to coat evenly. Add tomatoes and hearts of palm and toss gently.

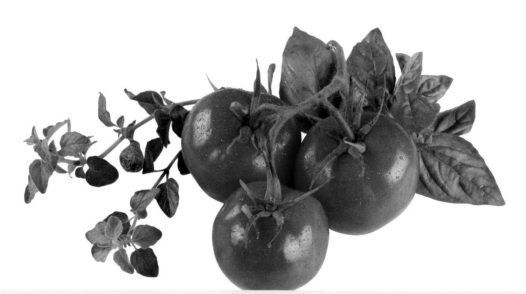

Calories 100	Cholesterol 0 mg	
Calories from fat 55	Sodium 310 mg	**EXCHANGES PER SERVING**
Total fat 6.0 g	Total carbohydrate 9 g	2 vegetable
Saturated fat 0.4 g	Dietary fiber 2 g	1 fat
Trans fat 0.0 g	Sugars 7 g	
	Protein 3 g	

SWEET AND CRISPY CUCUMBER-ANAHEIM SALAD

YIELD 4 servings | **SERVING SIZE** ¾ cup

This dish offers both good looks and personality. Its heat is mild enough for anyone to enjoy.

SALAD

- 1 medium Anaheim chile pepper
- 1 large cucumber, peeled and sliced
- ½ cup thinly sliced red onion

VINAIGRETTE

- ¼ cup white wine vinegar
- 3 tablespoons pourable sugar substitute
- 1 tablespoon canola oil
- ¼ teaspoon salt
- ¼ teaspoon coarsely ground black pepper

1 Slice pepper into thin rounds. For a milder dish, discard seeds and membranes. Combine pepper rounds, cucumber, and onion in a medium bowl.

2 In a small jar, combine all vinaigrette ingredients. Secure lid and shake vigorously until well blended. Pour over cucumber mixture. Toss gently, yet thoroughly, to blend. Let stand 15 minutes before serving.

		EXCHANGES PER SERVING
Calories 65	Cholesterol 0 mg	
Calories from fat 30	Sodium 150 mg	1 vegetable
Total fat 3.5 g	Total carbohydrate 6 g	1 fat
Saturated fat 0.3 g	Dietary fiber 1 g	
Trans fat 0.0 g	Sugars 4 g	
	Protein 1 g	

Flavorful tip Anaheim chile peppers are readily available in major supermarkets. They are usually medium green in color and have a long, narrow shape. They are the mildest of the chiles, but contain some heat.

BARLEY-ARTICHOKE SALAD ON ROMAINE

YIELD 4 servings | **SERVING SIZE** ¾ cup

Barley is the star in this dish. It acts like pasta—filling and energizing. Black, green, and red vegetables support the barley with bold color and freshness.

2 cups water

½ cup dried quick-cooking barley

½ of 13.75-ounce can quartered artichoke hearts, drained and coarsely chopped

8 small pitted ripe olives, chopped

1 medium tomato, seeded and diced

1 cup loosely packed fresh spinach, coarsely chopped

2 tablespoons chopped fresh basil leaves or ¼ cup chopped fresh parsley leaves

2 tablespoons red wine vinegar

1 tablespoon canola oil

¼ teaspoon salt

4 medium romaine leaves, rinsed and patted dry

1 Bring water to a boil in a medium saucepan over high heat. Add barley and return to a boil. Reduce heat and simmer, covered tightly, 10 minutes or until tender.

2 Meanwhile, in a medium bowl, combine remaining ingredients, except lettuce leaves.

3 Drain cooked barley in a colander, run under cold water to cool quickly, and shake off excess liquid. Place in a bowl with the artichoke mixture and toss gently, yet thoroughly, to blend. Serve equal amounts on each lettuce leaf.

Calories 135	Cholesterol 0 mg	**EXCHANGES PER SERVING**
Calories from fat 40	Sodium 335 mg	
Total fat 4.5 g	Total carbohydrate 21 g	1 starch
Saturated fat 0.4 g	Dietary fiber 4 g	1 vegetable
Trans fat 0.0 g	Sugars 2 g	1 fat
	Protein 3 g	

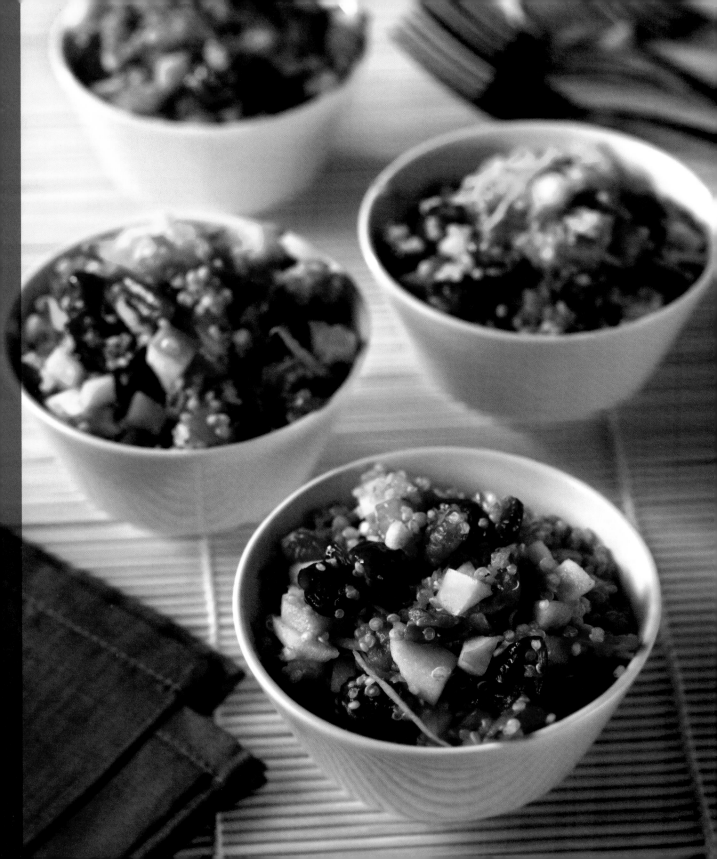

QUINOA AND BROWNED ONION SALAD
with Apples

YIELD 4 servings | **SERVING SIZE** ³⁄₄ cup

If you've never had browned onions in a salad, this is the time to try it. The onions are sweet and nutty and bring out the flavor of the pecans.

2 cups water

½ cup dried quinoa

¼ cup (1 ounce) pecan pieces

1 tablespoon plus 1 teaspoon canola oil, divided

1 cup finely chopped red onions

1 cup finely chopped Granny Smith apple

¼ cup dried cranberries or cherries

2 tablespoons balsamic vinegar

1 tablespoon pourable sugar substitute

½ teaspoon orange zest

¼ teaspoon salt

⅛ teaspoon dried red pepper flakes

1 Bring water to boil in a medium saucepan over high heat. Add quinoa and return to a boil. Reduce heat and simmer, covered tightly, 10 minutes or until liquid is absorbed. Drain in a fine-mesh sieve and run under cold water to cool quickly, shaking off excess liquid.

2 Meanwhile, heat a medium nonstick skillet over medium-high heat. Add nuts and cook 2–3 minutes or until lightly browned, stirring frequently. Remove from skillet and set aside.

3 Heat 1 teaspoon canola oil in the skillet, tilting to coat bottom lightly. Add onions and cook 8 minutes or until richly browned, stirring frequently. Remove from heat and set aside on a dinner plate in a thin layer to cool quickly, about 4 minutes.

4 Combine remaining ingredients in a medium bowl. Add quinoa, onions, and nuts, tossing gently, yet thoroughly, until well blended.

Fresh tip Quinoa is an excellent vegetarian source of protein. It is gluten-free and a good source of fiber and minerals as well. If not available, quinoa may be substituted with brown rice.

		EXCHANGES PER SERVING
Calories 240	Cholesterol 0 mg	1 starch
Calories from fat 100	Sodium 150 mg	½ fruit
Total fat 11.0 g	Total carbohydrate 33 g	1 vegetable
Saturated fat 1.0 g	Dietary fiber 4 g	2 fat
Trans fat 0.0 g	Sugars 13 g	
	Protein 4 g	

ASPARAGUS-WHEAT BERRY SALAD
with Blue Cheese

YIELD 5 servings | **SERVING SIZE** ½ cup

Wheat berries are new to many North Americans, but they've been around for at least 6,000 years. They add a crunchy texture to this salad, along with fiber.

½ cup dried wheat berries

3 cups water

6 fresh asparagus spears, trimmed and cut into 1-inch pieces

½ cup chopped fresh parsley leaves

1½ teaspoons fresh rosemary leaves, chopped, or ½ teaspoon dried rosemary leaves, crumbled

1 teaspoon lemon zest

1 tablespoon fresh lemon juice

1 tablespoon canola oil

¼ teaspoon salt

¼ cup (1 ounce) reduced-fat blue cheese, crumbled

1 Bring wheat berries and water to a boil in a large saucepan over high heat. Reduce heat, cover, and simmer 50 minutes or until tender.

2 Add asparagus to wheat berries in saucepan, cover, and cook 2–3 minutes or until just tender crisp. Drain wheat berry mixture in a fine-mesh strainer and run under cold water to cool quickly. Shake off excess liquid and place in a medium bowl. Add remaining ingredients, except cheese. Toss gently, yet thoroughly, until well blended. Add cheese and toss gently.

Calories 110
Calories from fat 40
Total fat 4.5 g
Saturated fat 1.0 g
Trans fat 0.0 g

Cholesterol 5 mg
Sodium 200 mg
Total carbohydrate 14 g
Dietary fiber 3 g
Sugars 0 g
Protein 5 g

EXCHANGES PER SERVING
1 starch
½ fat

Fast tip If desired, cook the wheat berries 24 hours in advance and store them in the refrigerator until needed. Assemble the salad ingredients at the time of serving or no longer than 30 minutes ahead for peak flavors and texture.

WILTED KALE SALAD

Kale—a dark green, ruffled form of cabbage—is the new rage among foodies and it's great for you, too!

VINAIGRETTE

¼ cup water

2–3 tablespoons cider vinegar

1 tablespoon sugar

2 teaspoons canola oil

⅛ teaspoon salt (optional)

SALAD

2 teaspoons canola oil, divided

1 cup finely chopped smoked turkey sausage

½ cup chopped onion

¼ of 16-ounce package fresh kale, coarsely chopped, washed well, and patted dry

8 tomato slices (optional)

Louisiana-style hot sauce, to taste

1 Combine vinaigrette ingredients in a jar, secure lid, and shake vigorously to blend well.

2 Heat 1 teaspoon canola oil in a large nonstick skillet over medium-high heat. Tilt skillet to coat bottom lightly; add sausage and cook 3 minutes or until browned, stirring frequently. Set aside on a separate plate.

3 Add remaining 1 teaspoon canola oil, tilt skillet, add onion, and cook 3 minutes, stirring frequently. Add kale, sausage, and vinaigrette; cook 30 seconds, stirring constantly with two utensils. Place on top of tomato slices and sprinkle with desired amount of hot sauce. Serve immediately for peak flavors.

Fresh tip You can make this salad with any kind of greens—from mustard to spinach. Canola oil, which is light in color, texture, and taste, is ideal for vinaigrettes that accompany greens, vegetables, fruit salads, and refreshing slaws.

Calories 85	Cholesterol 15 mg
Calories from fat 45	Sodium 175 mg
Total fat 5.0 g	Total carbohydrate 6 g
Saturated fat 0.9 g	Dietary fiber 1 g
Trans fat 0.0 g	Sugars 3 g
	Protein 3 g

EXCHANGES PER SERVING
½ carbohydrate
1 fat

SPINACH SALAD
with Grilled and Fresh Fruit

YIELD 4 servings | **SERVING SIZE** 1¾ cups

Serving grilled fruit with fresh fruit not only makes a great-looking combination, but also provides two layers of flavor.

Canola oil cooking spray

¼ cup raspberry blush vinegar

1 tablespoon sugar

1 tablespoon canola oil

1–2 teaspoons grated fresh ginger

2 slices fresh pineapple, about ½-inch thick, or two medium peaches, pitted and halved

4 cups loosely packed spinach

¼ cup thinly sliced red onion

1 cup quartered strawberries

1 Coat grill or grill pan with cooking spray and place over medium-high heat.

2 Combine vinegar, sugar, canola oil, and ginger in a small jar, secure lid tightly, and shake vigorously until completely blended. Place pineapple slices or peach halves on plate; drizzle 1 tablespoon vinegar mixture evenly over both sides.

3 Place pineapple or peaches on grill rack and grill 4 minutes or until soft and slightly browned. Turn and cook 4 minutes or until heated through. Cut fruit into bite-size pieces.

4 Place spinach and onion on a serving platter. Top with grilled fruit, sprinkle strawberries evenly on top, and drizzle remaining dressing over all.

Calories 95
Calories from fat 30
Total fat 3.5 g
Saturated fat 0.3 g
Trans fat 0.0 g
Cholesterol 0 mg
Sodium 15 mg
Total carbohydrate 16 g
Dietary fiber 2 g
Sugars 11 g
Protein 1 g

EXCHANGES PER SERVING
1 fruit
½ fat

Fresh tip Be creative on the grill. Try nectarines, pears, or even orange slices. Brushing the fruits with a little canola oil will prevent them from sticking to the grill. If raspberry blush vinegar is unavailable, regular raspberry vinegar may be substituted.

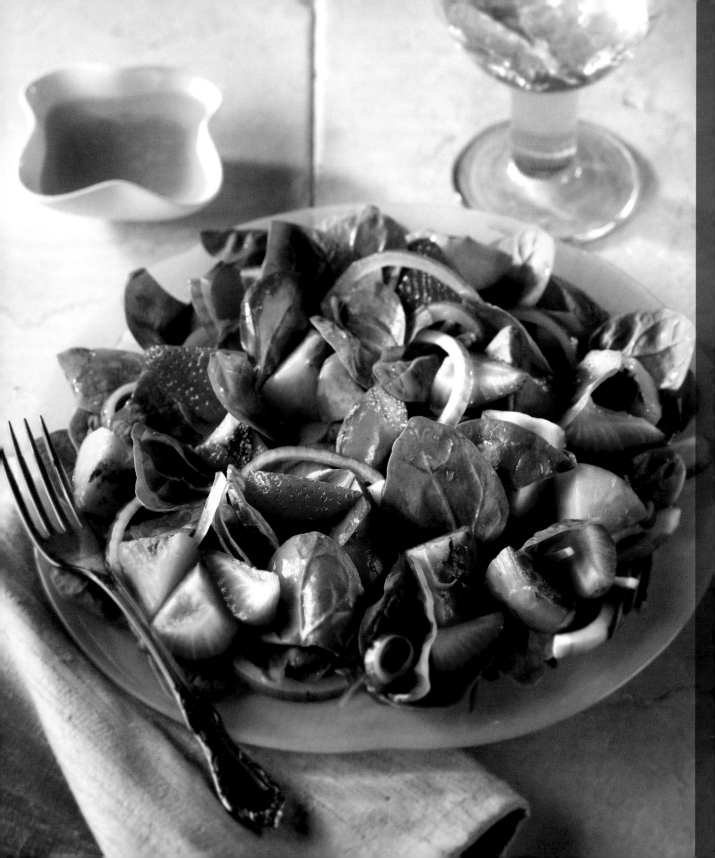

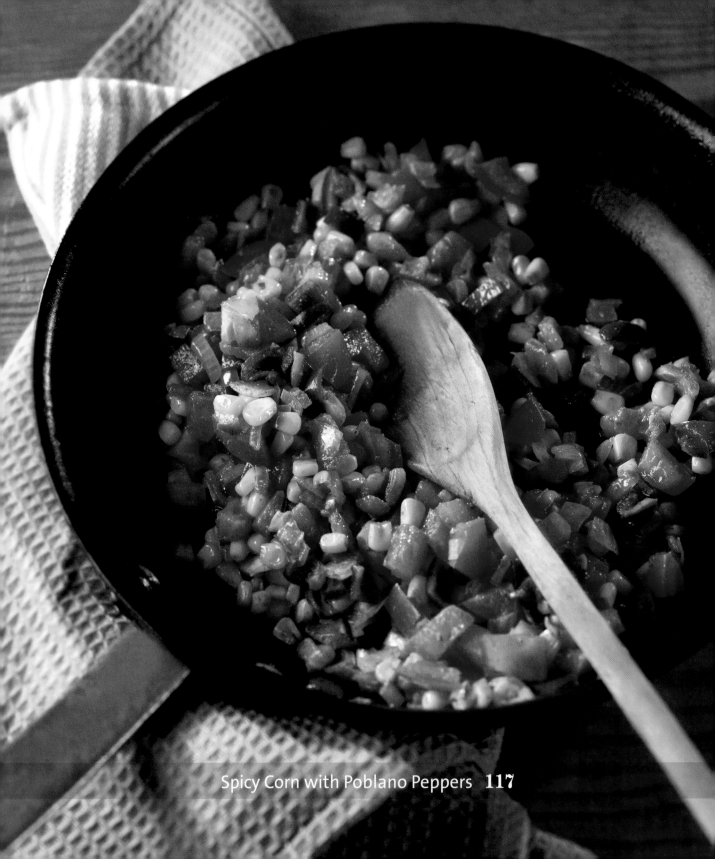

Spicy Corn with Poblano Peppers **117**

SIDES

Asparagus with Creamy Dijon Sauce | 112

Black Beans with Green Chile Sauce | 113

Black-Eyed Peas with Jalapeño and
   Tomatoes | 114

Skillet Broccoli with Tangy Sweet Sauce | 116

Spicy Corn with Poblano Peppers | 117

Stewed Eggplant, Tomatoes, and
   Fresh Basil | 118

Green Beans with Spicy Mustard Sauce | 119

Turnip Greens with Smoked Sausage | 120

Cumin'd Lentils and Carrots | 121

Garlic Snow Peas with Cilantro | 123

Crispy Crunchy Oven-Fried Okra | 124

Stuffed Portobello Caps with Parmesan
   Crumb Topping | 125

Baked Acorn Squash with Cranberry-Orange
   Sauce | 126

Toasted Sesame Seed Quinoa | 128

Yellow Rice and Red Pepper Tosser | 129

Spinach and Mushroom Barley Pilaf | 130

Roasted Root Vegetables with Balsamic
   Reduction | 132

Sweet Potatoes with Caramelized
   Sherry Onions | 133

Zucchini Boats | 134

High-Roasted Onions | 135

ASPARAGUS WITH CREAMY DIJON SAUCE

YIELD 4 servings | **SERVING SIZE** 6 asparagus spears

Add zip to asparagus without the fat or calories of traditional cream sauces.

Canola oil cooking spray

24 asparagus spears, ends trimmed (about 1 lb)

2 tablespoons coarse-grain Dijon mustard

2 tablespoons fat-free sour cream

1 tablespoon canola mayonnaise

2 teaspoons fresh lemon juice (optional)

2 tablespoons fat-free milk

¼ teaspoon dried tarragon leaves

¼–½ teaspoon coarsely ground black pepper

1 Preheat oven to 425°F.

2 Place asparagus on a large foil-lined baking sheet coated with cooking spray. Coat asparagus evenly with spray, roll back and forth to coat evenly, and roast 12 minutes or until tender crisp.

3 Meanwhile, whisk together remaining ingredients, except black pepper, in a small saucepan. Place over medium heat 1–2 minutes or until thoroughly heated. Do not bring to a boil. Remove from heat, place asparagus on a serving platter, and spoon sauce down center. Top with black pepper.

		EXCHANGES PER SERVING
Calories 45	Cholesterol 0 mg	
Calories from fat 15	Sodium 225 mg	1 vegetable
Total fat 1.5 g	Total carbohydrate 6 g	½ fat
Saturated fat 0.1 g	Dietary fiber 2 g	
Trans fat 0.0 g	Sugars 2 g	
	Protein 3 g	

Flavorful tip Coarse-grain Dijon contains mustard seeds, which add a nice texture to this dish. If desired, substitute regular Dijon for an even creamier sauce.

BLACK BEANS
with Green Chile Sauce

YIELD 4 servings | SERVING SIZE ½ cup

Wake up beans with this tangy tomato and salsa verde topping. This dish can also be served as a meatless entrée over brown rice or in a tortilla.

1 tablespoon canola oil, divided

1 cup diced onions

2 medium cloves garlic, minced

½ teaspoon ground cumin

½ cup water

1 can (15 ounces) no-salt-added black beans, rinsed and drained

½ cup diced tomato

¼ cup salsa verde

1 Heat 1 teaspoon canola oil in a large nonstick skillet over medium-high heat. Add onions and cook 3 minutes. Add garlic and cumin and cook 30 seconds. Add water, beans, and tomato. Bring just to a boil, reduce heat, cover, and simmer 5 minutes.

2 Meanwhile, in a small bowl, combine salsa verde with remaining 2 teaspoons canola oil. Serve beans topped with salsa verde mixture.

Flavorful tip Adding canola oil to the salsa verde cuts the acidity in the dish in the same way that adding canola oil to a vinaigrette reduces its sharpness.

Calories 145
  Calories from fat 35
Total fat 4.0 g
  Saturated fat 0.4 g
  Trans fat 0.0 g

Cholesterol 0 mg
Sodium 55 mg
Total carbohydrate 23 g
  Dietary fiber 5 g
  Sugars 4 g
Protein 6 g

EXCHANGES PER SERVING
1 starch
1 vegetable
1 fat

BLACK-EYED PEAS
with Jalapeño and Tomatoes

YIELD 4 servings | **SERVING SIZE** ½ cup

Black-eyed peas are generally cooked with bacon, but you won't miss it in this recipe because of the seasonings. It's "thyme" to enjoy these peas without bacon.

1 tablespoon canola oil

1 cup diced onions

1 medium jalapeño, cut into thinly sliced rounds (with seeds)

1 cup water

1 package (10 ounces) frozen black-eyed peas

1 tablespoon cider vinegar, divided

¼ teaspoon dried thyme leaves

½ cup diced tomato

½ teaspoon salt

1 Heat canola oil in a large saucepan over medium-high heat. Immediately reduce heat to medium, add onions and jalapeño, and cook 3–4 minutes or until beginning to turn golden. Add water; bring to a boil over high heat. Add peas, 1 teaspoon vinegar, and thyme. Return to a boil.

2 Reduce heat and simmer, covered, 25 minutes or until peas are tender. Remove from heat and add tomato, remaining 2 teaspoons vinegar, and salt.

Calories 155
   Calories from fat 35
Total fat 4.0 g
   Saturated fat 0.4 g
   Trans fat 0.0 g

Cholesterol 0 mg
Sodium 305 mg
Total carbohydrate 24 g
   Dietary fiber 5 g
   Sugars 4 g
Protein 7 g

EXCHANGES PER SERVING
1 starch
1 vegetable
1 fat

Fresh tip Wearing gloves when handling jalapeños or other hot peppers protects your hands and eyes from coming into contact with pepper substances that can cause a burning sensation.

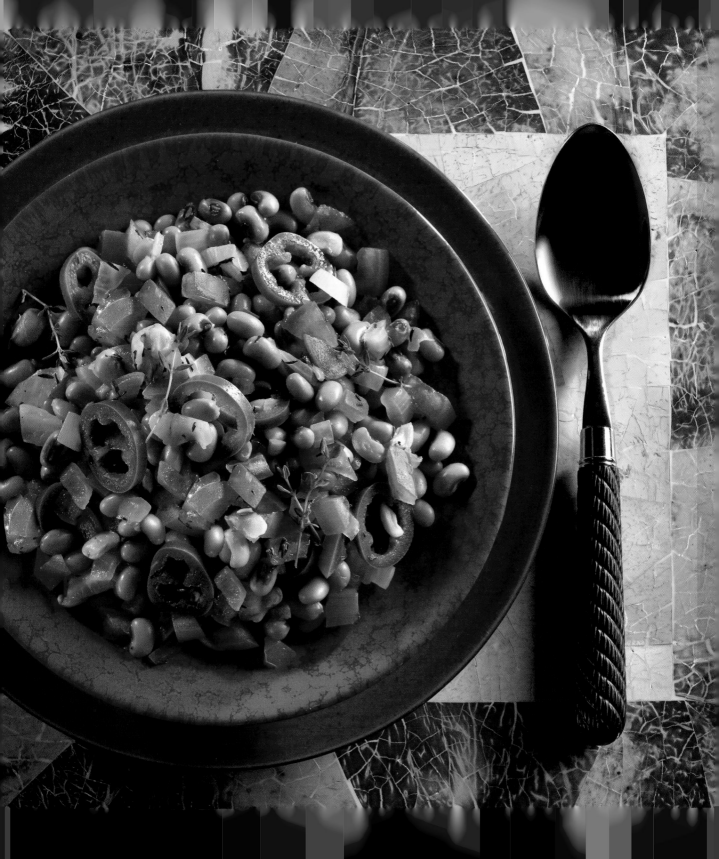

SKILLET BROCCOLI
with Tangy Sweet Sauce

YIELD 4 servings | **SERVING SIZE** 1 cup

Want a change from steaming broccoli? Try skillet-roasting! It gives broccoli a rustic appeal.

1 tablespoon canola oil

4 cups (12 ounces) fresh broccoli florets

SAUCE

1½ tablespoons balsamic vinegar

2 teaspoons sugar

¼ teaspoon salt

⅛–¼ teaspoon dried red pepper flakes

1 Heat a large nonstick skillet over medium heat, add canola oil, and swirl until well coated. Add broccoli, cover, and cook 10 minutes or until lightly browned and tender crisp, stirring frequently.

2 Meanwhile, combine sauce ingredients in a small bowl and set aside. Remove skillet from heat. Add sauce and toss gently, yet thoroughly, to blend.

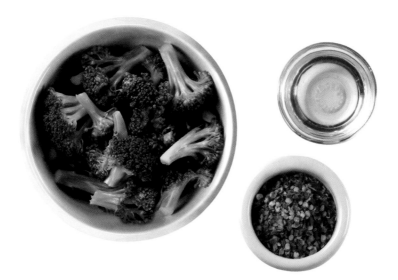

Calories 65
    Calories from fat 35
Total fat 4.0 g
    Saturated fat 0.3 g
    Trans fat 0.0 g

Cholesterol 0 mg
Sodium 170 mg
Total carbohydrate 8 g
    Dietary fiber 2 g
    Sugars 5 g
Protein 3 g

EXCHANGES PER SERVING
1 vegetable
½ fat

Fast tip Keeping the broccoli covered while skillet-roasting it in canola oil steams and sautés it at the same time, without adding water. This unique technique also works well with other vegetables, such as carrots and potatoes.

Enjoy this dish for a quick trip to Mexico!

1 tablespoon canola oil

1 medium poblano pepper, stemmed, seeded, and chopped

1 cup diced onions

1½ cups frozen corn, thawed

1 teaspoon chili powder

½ teaspoon ground cumin

½ medium tomato, seeded and diced

½ teaspoon salt

1 Heat canola oil in a large nonstick skillet over medium-high heat. Add pepper and onions and cook 6 minutes or until very richly browned, stirring frequently. Stir in corn, chili powder, and cumin; sauté 1 minute.

2 Remove from heat; add tomato and salt. Toss gently. Let stand 2 minutes to absorb flavors and bring out moisture. Stir before serving.

Flavorful tip Be sure to seed the tomato, or the dish's rich flavors will be diluted by the tomato juice. However, if you want more heat, leave in the pepper seeds.

Calories 100	Cholesterol 0 mg	**EXCHANGES PER SERVING**
Calories from fat 35	Sodium 300 mg	½ starch
Total fat 4.0 g	Total carbohydrate 17 g	1 vegetable
Saturated fat 0.3 g	Dietary fiber 3 g	1 fat
Trans fat 0.0 g	Sugars 5 g	
	Protein 2 g	

STEWED EGGPLANT, TOMATOES, AND FRESH BASIL

YIELD 6 servings | **SERVING SIZE** ⅔ cup

Stewing over what to pair with your Italian-inspired entrée? Try this unbeatable combination of vegetables and seasonings. That's amore!

1 tablespoon canola oil

1 cup diced onions

1 cup chopped green bell pepper

2 medium cloves garlic, minced

1 medium eggplant (about 8 ounces), cut into ½-inch cubes

1 small zucchini, thinly sliced

1 can (14.5 ounces) stewed tomatoes with Italian seasonings

2–4 tablespoons chopped fresh basil leaves

1 teaspoon sugar

¼ teaspoon salt

1 Heat canola oil in a large saucepan over medium-high heat. Add onions and pepper; cook 4 minutes or until onions are translucent. Add garlic and cook 15 seconds. Stir in eggplant, zucchini, and tomatoes. Bring to a boil, reduce heat, cover, and simmer 10 minutes.

2 Remove from heat and add basil, sugar, and salt. Let stand 10 minutes to absorb flavors.

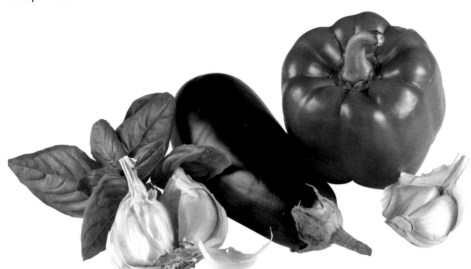

Calories 75
  Calories from fat 20
Total fat 2.5 g
  Saturated fat 0.2 g
  Trans fat 0.0 g

Cholesterol 0 mg
Sodium 295 mg
Total carbohydrate 12 g
  Dietary fiber 3 g
  Sugars 7 g
Protein 2 g

EXCHANGES PER SERVING
2 vegetable
½ fat

Flavorful tip Fresh herbs should always be added at the end of cooking for peak flavors. Dried herbs need time to release their flavors, so add them during the cooking time or crush them between your fingertips to release the flavors.

GREEN BEANS WITH SPICY MUSTARD SAUCE

YIELD 6 servings | **SERVING SIZE** ²⁄₃ cup

This aromatic bowl of fresh beans will dress up the simplest of dinners.

2 cups water

4 cups (1 lb) green beans, stems removed

SAUCE

1 tablespoon canola oil

1½ tablespoons coarse-grain Dijon mustard

1 teaspoon Louisiana-style hot sauce

¼ teaspoon salt

2 teaspoons sesame seeds, toasted (optional)

1 Place 2 cups water in a large saucepan with a collapsible steamer basket. Place green beans on top of basket. Bring to a boil over high heat. Cover tightly and steam 7–8 minutes or until tender crisp.

2 Meanwhile, combine sauce ingredients in a small bowl.

3 Place green beans in a serving bowl, add sauce, and toss gently to coat lightly. Sprinkle with sesame seeds.

Fresh tip If you don't have a steamer basket, boil the beans in a large covered saucepan with 1 cup water for the same amount of time. Be sure to drain them well.

Calories 45	Cholesterol 0 mg
Calories from fat 20	Sodium 195 mg
Total fat 2.5 g	Total carbohydrate 6 g
Saturated fat 0.2 g	Dietary fiber 2 g
Trans fat 0.0 g	Sugars 1 g
	Protein 1 g

EXCHANGES PER SERVING

1 vegetable

½ fat

TURNIP GREENS WITH SMOKED SAUSAGE

YIELD 8 servings | **SERVING SIZE** ½ cup

Here's a "healthified" Southern classic using browned turkey sausage instead of bacon for less fat but all the flavor.

3 teaspoons canola oil, divided

1 cup (¼ lb) low-fat smoked turkey sausage, diced

6 cups water

1 cup chopped onions

1 tablespoon cider vinegar

2 teaspoons sugar

1 bag (16 ounces) fresh turnip greens

¾ teaspoon salt

    Louisiana-style hot sauce (optional)

1 Heat 1 teaspoon canola oil in a Dutch oven over medium-high heat. Tilt Dutch oven to coat bottom lightly. Add sausage and cook until browned, stirring frequently. Set aside on a separate plate.

2 Add water, onions, vinegar, and sugar to the Dutch oven and bring to a boil over high heat. Gradually add turnip greens, bring to a boil, and stir until wilted. Reduce heat, cover, and simmer 30 minutes or until tender. Drain greens, reserving ½ cup liquid. Return drained greens to Dutch oven along with reserved liquid, sausage, remaining 2 teaspoons canola oil, and salt. Let stand 5 minutes to absorb flavors. Serve with hot sauce.

Calories 65
  Calories from fat 25
Total fat 3.0 g
  Saturated fat 0.7 g
  Trans fat 0.0 g

Cholesterol 10 mg
Sodium 365 mg
Total carbohydrate 6 g
  Dietary fiber 2 g
  Sugars 1 g
Protein 3 g

EXCHANGES PER SERVING
1 vegetable
½ fat

Flavorful tip Just a small amount of browned sausage is all you need to give a meaty taste to a "mess of greens."

CUMIN'D LENTILS AND CARROTS

This dish offers a bang for your buck and for your health. Canola oil has half the saturated fat of olive oil for a fraction of the price. Lentils and carrots offer essential nutrients for less than a dollar per serving.

1½ tablespoons canola oil, divided
1 cup diced carrots
1 cup diced onions
1¼ cups water
⅓ cup dried lentils
½ teaspoon ground cumin, divided
½ teaspoon salt
½ teaspoon sugar

1 Heat 1 tablespoon canola oil in a large nonstick skillet over medium-high heat. Cook carrots and onions 8 minutes or until richly browned, stirring frequently. Add water, lentils, and ¼ teaspoon cumin. Bring to a boil, reduce heat, cover tightly, and simmer 25 minutes or until lentils are tender.

2 Remove from heat and add remaining ingredients.

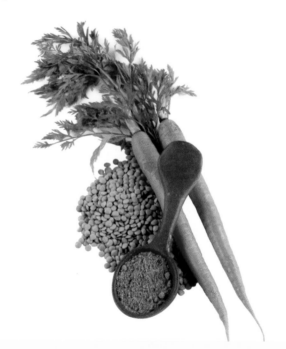

Calories 130
  Calories from fat 55
Total fat 6.0 g
  Saturated fat 0.4 g
  Trans fat 0.0 g

Cholesterol 0 mg
Sodium 315 mg
Total carbohydrate 17 g
  Dietary fiber 5 g
  Sugars 4 g
Protein 5 g

EXCHANGES PER SERVING
½ starch
1 vegetable
1 fat

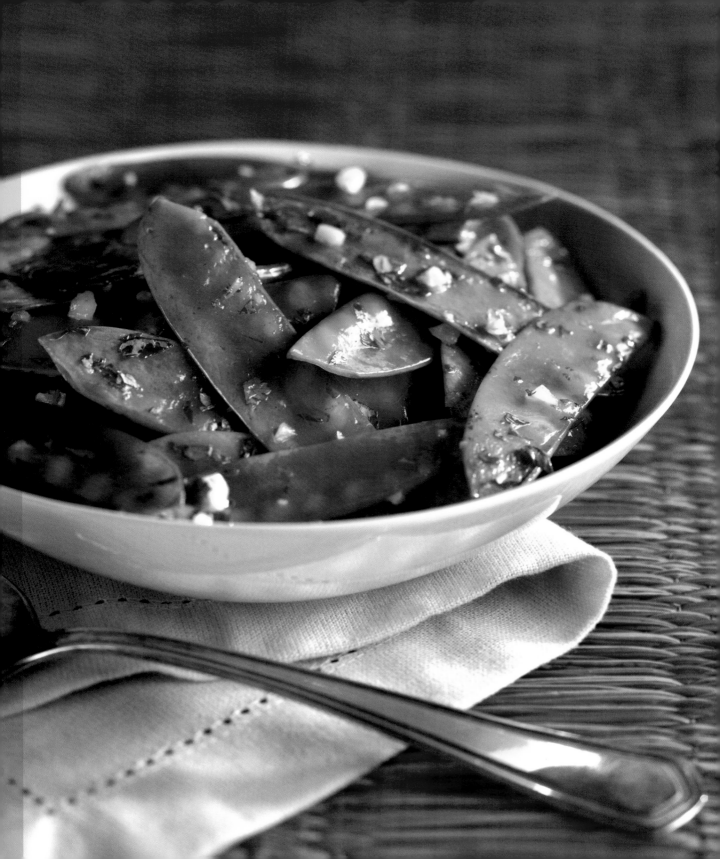

GARLIC SNOW PEAS WITH CILANTRO

YIELD 6 servings | **SERVING SIZE** ½ cup

Ready in less than 5 minutes, this oh-so-simple side dish is perfect for the busiest of days.

3 teaspoons canola oil, divided

3 cups fresh (or frozen and thawed) snow peas, patted dry and trimmed

4 medium cloves garlic, minced

¼ teaspoon salt

¼–½ cup chopped fresh cilantro leaves

1 Working in two batches, heat 1½ teaspoons canola oil in a large nonstick skillet over medium-high heat. Add half of the snow peas; cook 3 minutes or until just beginning to brown on edges, using two utensils to toss easily. Add half of garlic and cook 30 seconds, stirring constantly. Set aside on a separate plate.

2 Repeat with remaining 1½ teaspoons canola oil, snow peas, and garlic. When cooked, return the reserved snow peas to skillet; add salt and cilantro and toss gently, yet thoroughly. Serve immediately for peak flavors.

Calories 45
 Calories from fat 20
Total fat 2.5 g
 Saturated fat 0.2 g
 Trans fat 0.0 g

Cholesterol 0 mg
Sodium 100 mg
Total carbohydrate 4 g
 Dietary fiber 2 g
 Sugars 2 g
Protein 2 g

EXCHANGES PER SERVING
1 vegetable
½ fat

CRISPY CRUNCHY OVEN-FRIED OKRA

YIELD 7 servings | **SERVING SIZE** ½ cup

These okra bites are so crunchy and tasty that you'll want to eat them like popcorn. Put a little "South" in your mouth!

Canola oil cooking spray

¾ cup low-fat buttermilk

1 tablespoon Louisiana-style hot sauce

2 cups fresh okra, trimmed and cut into ½-inch rounds

¾ cup yellow cornmeal

1 teaspoon paprika

¼ teaspoon garlic powder (optional)

¼ teaspoon black pepper

¾ teaspoon salt, divided

1½ tablespoons canola oil

1 Preheat oven 475°F. Lightly coat a large, foil-lined baking sheet with cooking spray and set aside.

2 Combine buttermilk and hot sauce in a medium bowl; add okra and toss to coat evenly. Let stand 10 minutes.

3 Meanwhile, place remaining ingredients, except ½ teaspoon salt and canola oil, in a shallow pan, such as a pie pan, and mix well.

4 Working in small batches, remove okra from buttermilk mixture and coat it evenly with cornmeal mixture. Place on the baking sheet in a single layer, being careful to leave space between pieces. Drizzle canola oil evenly over all and bake 10–11 minutes or until golden brown on the bottom. Remove from oven and sprinkle with remaining ½ teaspoon salt.

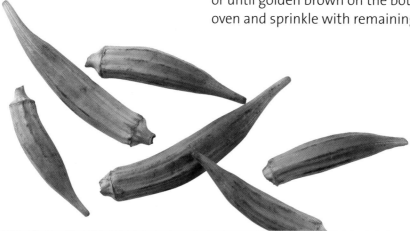

Calories 105
    Calories from fat 30
Total fat 3.5 g
    Saturated fat 0.4 g
    Trans fat 0.0 g

Cholesterol 0 mg
Sodium 295 mg
Total carbohydrate 16 g
    Dietary fiber 2 g
    Sugars 2 g
Protein 3 g

EXCHANGES PER SERVING
1 starch
½ fat

Flavorful tip Drizzling canola oil over the okra pieces makes for even browning.

STUFFED PORTOBELLO CAPS
with Parmesan Crumb Topping

YIELD 4 servings | **SERVING SIZE** 1 portobello cap

The mushrooms are so good and filling, you could almost make a meal of them alone, but they are best served beside a cut of pork, poultry, or fish for quick and simple protein.

4 medium Portobello caps, wiped clean with a damp towel and gills removed (by gently scraping with the tip of a spoon)

2 tablespoons balsamic vinegar

4 teaspoons canola oil, divided

1/2 teaspoon garlic salt

Canola oil cooking spray

1 small zucchini, diced

1/2 cup diced green bell pepper

1/2 teaspoon dried oregano leaves

1/4 cup diced roasted red peppers

1/4 cup panko bread crumbs

1/4 cup (1 ounce) grated Parmesan cheese

1 Preheat oven to 425°F. Place mushrooms on a foil-lined baking sheet. Combine vinegar, 2 teaspoons canola oil, and garlic salt in a small container. Brush mixture evenly over both sides of mushrooms, turning and brushing until all is applied. Turn mushrooms stem side down and bake 10 minutes.

2 Meanwhile, heat a large nonstick skillet over medium-high heat. Coat with cooking spray. Add zucchini, bell pepper, and oregano. Lightly coat vegetables with cooking spray and cook 6–7 minutes or until zucchini is just tender and browned, stirring frequently. Remove from heat.

3 Remove mushrooms from oven, turn over, and top with equal amounts of roasted peppers and zucchini mixture. Combine bread crumbs and Parmesan in a small bowl. Spoon equal amounts over each mushroom; drizzle remaining 2 teaspoons canola oil evenly over all. Bake 7 minutes or until lightly golden. Remove and let stand 5 minutes for peak flavor and texture.

Flavorful tip Let the mushrooms stand 5 minutes before serving to allow their flavors to absorb. This makes a difference in their overall taste and texture.

Calories 110	Cholesterol 5 mg	
Calories from fat 65	Sodium 235 mg	**EXCHANGES PER SERVING**
Total fat 7.0 g	Total carbohydrate 9 g	2 vegetable
Saturated fat 1.4 g	Dietary fiber 1 g	1 1/2 fat
Trans fat 0.0 g	Sugars 4 g	
	Protein 5 g	

BAKED ACORN SQUASH
with Cranberry-Orange Sauce

YIELD 4 servings | **SERVING SIZE** 1 squash quarter

Harvest the colors and flavors of fall in this pretty side dish. It is a great replacement for heavier dishes like green bean or sweet potato casseroles.

Canola oil cooking spray

¼ cup dried cranberries

1 teaspoon orange zest

¼ cup orange juice

1 tablespoon canola oil

1 large acorn squash (about 1½ lbs), quartered lengthwise, seeded, and skin pierced with a fork in several places

1–2 tablespoons brown sugar substitute

⅛ teaspoon salt

1 teaspoon vanilla

1 Preheat oven to 375°F. Lightly coat a 9-inch, deep-dish pie pan or baking dish with cooking spray. In the pan, stir together cranberries, zest, juice, and canola oil. Place squash cut side down on top of cranberry mixture. Cover with foil and bake 45 minutes or until tender crisp when pierced with a fork. Turn each piece to other cut side down; bake uncovered 15 minutes or until squash is tender.

2 Remove squash and place on a serving plate. Add brown sugar substitute, salt, and vanilla to cranberry mixture; spoon equal amounts of mixture on each piece of squash.

Calories 130	Cholesterol 0 mg	**EXCHANGES PER SERVING**
Calories from fat 35	Sodium 80 mg	
Total fat 4.0 g	Total carbohydrate 25 g	1 starch
Saturated fat 0.3 g	Dietary fiber 5 g	½ fruit
Trans fat 0.0 g	Sugars 14 g	½ fat
	Protein 1 g	

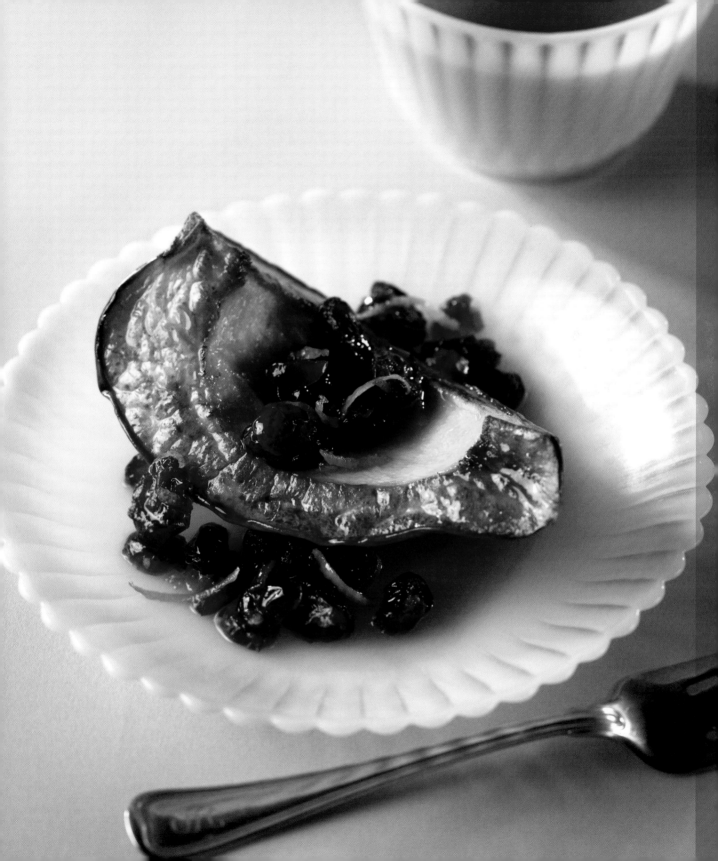

TOASTED SESAME SEED QUINOA

YIELD 6 servings | **SERVING SIZE** ½ cup

Quinoa has a bit of crunch to it and when tossed with toasted sesame seeds, it takes on a slightly nutty flavor.

1½ cups water
¾ cup quick-cooking quinoa
½ teaspoon curry powder
⅛ teaspoon cayenne pepper (optional)
½ cup golden raisins
1 tablespoon sesame seeds
2 tablespoons canola oil, divided
1 cup diced onions
1 cup diced red bell pepper
¼ teaspoon salt

1 Bring water to a boil in a medium saucepan over high heat; add quinoa, curry powder, and cayenne pepper. Reduce heat, cover, and cook 7 minutes. Add raisins, cover, and continue to cook 3–4 minutes or until liquid is absorbed.

2 Meanwhile, heat a medium nonstick skillet over medium-high heat. Add sesame seeds; cook 1–2 minutes or until just beginning to brown, stirring constantly. Remove from skillet and set aside on a separate plate.

3 In the same skillet, heat 1 tablespoon canola oil over medium-high heat; add onions and cook 4 minutes or until beginning to richly brown. Add bell pepper and cook 2 minutes, stirring frequently.

4 Remove skillet from heat, add quinoa and salt, and toss to blend. Sprinkle evenly with sesame seeds and drizzle remaining canola oil over all. Do not stir.

Calories 155
Calories from fat 55
Total fat 6.0 g
Saturated fat 0.6 g
Trans fat 0.0 g

Cholesterol 0 mg
Sodium 105 mg
Total carbohydrate 23 g
Dietary fiber 3 g
Sugars 10 g
Protein 3 g

EXCHANGES PER SERVING
½ starch
½ fruit
1 vegetable
1 fat

Flavorful tip Not stirring in the canola oil allows it to pull out the richness of the other flavors, especially the sesame seeds.

YELLOW RICE AND RED PEPPER TOSSER

YIELD 4 servings | **SERVING SIZE** ½ cup

Turmeric gives this rice an inviting, brilliant yellow color, which complements other ingredient colors.

3 teaspoons canola oil, divided

½ cup diced onion

½ medium red bell pepper, thinly sliced and cut into 2-inch pieces

½ cup quick-cooking brown rice

1 cup water

⅛ teaspoon ground turmeric

½ of 1-ounce package taco seasoning mix

¼ cup chopped fresh cilantro leaves

1 medium lime, quartered

1 Heat 1 teaspoon canola oil in a large nonstick skillet over medium-high heat. Tilt skillet to coat bottom lightly. Add onion and cook 3 minutes or until brown on edges. Add another 1 teaspoon canola oil and bell pepper; cook 3 minutes, using two utensils to stir.

2 Add rice, water, and turmeric to skillet. Bring to a boil over medium-high heat. Reduce heat, cover, and simmer 10–12 minutes or until water is absorbed. Remove from heat; add taco seasoning, cilantro, and remaining 1 teaspoon canola oil. Toss gently and serve with fresh lime wedges.

Calories 140
  Calories from fat 35
Total fat 4.0 g
  Saturated fat 0.3 g
  Trans fat 0.0 g

Cholesterol 0 mg
Sodium 275 mg
Total carbohydrate 24 g
  Dietary fiber 2 g
  Sugars 2 g
Protein 3 g

EXCHANGES PER SERVING
1 starch
1 vegetable
1 fat

SPINACH AND MUSHROOM BARLEY PILAF

YIELD 4 servings | **SERVING SIZE** ½ cup

A dynamic duo in any dish, spinach and mushrooms have rustic textures and earthy flavors. This hearty side dish goes well with steak or pork.

1 cup water

½ cup quick-cooking barley

1½ tablespoons canola oil, divided

1½ cups diced onions

½ of 8-ounce package sliced mushrooms

2 medium cloves garlic, minced

2 cups (1 ounce) loosely packed baby spinach

1 teaspoon dried oregano leaves, crumbled

½ teaspoon salt

1 Bring water to a boil in a small saucepan over high heat. Stir in barley, reduce heat, cover tightly, and simmer 10–12 minutes or until tender. Remove from heat and let stand 5 minutes.

2 Meanwhile, heat ½ tablespoon canola oil in a large nonstick skillet over medium-high heat. Tilt skillet to coat bottom evenly; add onions, and cook 6 minutes or until richly browned, stirring frequently. Add mushrooms and cook 4 minutes or until tender, using two utensils to toss. Add garlic and cook 30 seconds, stirring constantly.

3 Remove from heat. Add spinach, oregano, salt, and undrained barley. Toss well to blend. Drizzle remaining 1 tablespoon canola oil evenly over all and toss gently until just coated.

Calories 150
Calories from fat 55
Total fat 6.0 g
Saturated fat 0.5 g
Trans fat 0.0 g

Cholesterol 0 mg
Sodium 300 mg
Total carbohydrate 24 g
Dietary fiber 4 g
Sugars 3 g
Protein 3 g

EXCHANGES PER SERVING
1 starch
1 vegetable
1 fat

Flavorful tip Do not drain the barley. The small amount of liquid that remains will add moisture to the dish without breaking down flavors. Add the remaining canola oil at the end for a smooth texture.

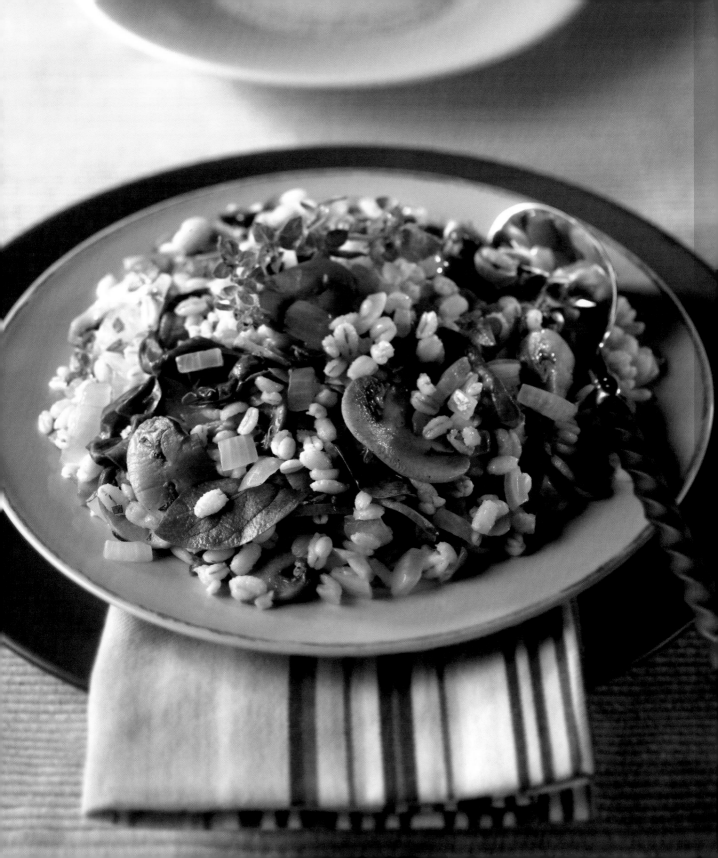

ROASTED ROOT VEGETABLES
with Balsamic Reduction

YIELD 4 servings | **SERVING SIZE** ½ cup

Reducing balsamic vinegar creates a syrupy, sweet sauce with a kick! And nothing says autumn better than roasted vegetables.

Canola oil cooking spray

2 medium beets, peeled and cut into ½-inch wedges

2 medium carrots, peeled, quartered lengthwise, and cut into 3-inch pieces

1 medium onion, cut into ½-inch wedges

1 tablespoon canola oil

¼ cup balsamic vinegar

¼ teaspoon salt

⅛ teaspoon black pepper

1 Preheat oven to 425°F. Line a baking sheet with foil, and lightly coat with cooking spray.

2 Place vegetables on the baking sheet, drizzle canola oil over all and toss gently, yet thoroughly, to coat evenly. Arrange in a single layer and bake 20 minutes or until vegetables are just tender and beginning to brown on the edges.

3 Remove from the oven. Bring vinegar to a boil in a small saucepan over medium-high heat. Boil for 1½–2 minutes or until liquid is reduced to 1 tablespoon. Place vegetables on a serving plate and drizzle reduction evenly over all. Sprinkle with salt and pepper.

Calories 85
Calories from fat 30
Total fat 3.5 g
Saturated fat 0.3 g
Trans fat 0.0 g

Cholesterol 0 mg
Sodium 195 mg
Total carbohydrate 14 g
Dietary fiber 2 g
Sugars 7 g
Protein 1 g

EXCHANGES PER SERVING
3 vegetable
½ fat

Fast tip To peel beets easily, use a vegetable peeler as you would for carrots.

SWEET POTATOES
with Caramelized Sherry Onions

YIELD 4 servings | **SERVING SIZE** 1 sweet potato

It doesn't take many ingredients for wonderful results! Try these flavor-packed sweet potatoes for something different with little fuss.

4 medium sweet potatoes (6 ounces each), pierced with fork in several areas

1 tablespoon canola oil

1½ cups very thinly sliced onions

2 teaspoons sugar

¼ cup dry sherry

1 teaspoon Worcestershire sauce

¼ teaspoon salt

1 Place potatoes in microwave and cook on high for 11 minutes or until fork-tender.

2 Meanwhile, heat canola oil in a large nonstick skillet over medium-high heat. Add onions and sugar. Cook 9–10 minutes or until very richly browned, stirring frequently. Add remaining ingredients and cook 30 seconds or until liquid is reduced slightly.

3 Split potatoes almost in half, fluff with a fork, and spoon equal amounts of onion mixture on each potato.

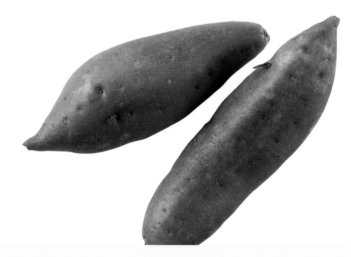

Flavorful tip Slice the onions extremely thin, so they will be richly browned and distribute the deep, sweet flavors of the other ingredients.

Calories 165
  Calories from fat 30
Total fat 3.5 g
  Saturated fat 0.3 g
  Trans fat 0.0 g

Cholesterol 0 mg
Sodium 200 mg
Total carbohydrate 29 g
  Dietary fiber 4 g
  Sugars 11 g
Protein 3 g

EXCHANGES PER SERVING
1½ starch
1 vegetable
½ fat

ZUCCHINI BOATS

YIELD 4 servings | **SERVING SIZE** 1 zucchini boat

*Give your zucchini an exciting new texture by having it act as a bowl
and filling it with bread crumbs and seasonings.*

2 medium zucchini, halved lengthwise

1 tablespoon canola oil, divided

1 cup finely chopped onions

1/2 teaspoon dried oregano leaves

1/2 cup panko bread crumbs, divided

1 egg white

1/2 teaspoon paprika

1/2 teaspoon salt

1/8 teaspoon cayenne pepper

1 Preheat oven to 375°F. Line a baking sheet with foil.

2 Using the tip of a teaspoon, scrape out the "meat" from the squash, creating four zucchini shells or boats. Coarsely chop "meat" of squash. Place shells on the baking sheet.

3 Heat 1 teaspoon canola oil in a large nonstick skillet over medium-high heat. Tilt skillet to coat bottom lightly. Add chopped zucchini, onions, and oregano and cook 4 minutes or until mixture begins to lightly brown, stirring frequently. Remove from heat and cool slightly (about 5 minutes).

4 Meanwhile, combine 1/4 cup bread crumbs with egg white, paprika, salt, and cayenne pepper in a small bowl. Add crumb mixture to slightly cooled squash mixture. Toss gently, yet thoroughly, to blend.

5 Fill shells with equal amounts of squash mixture. Sprinkle with remaining bread crumbs and drizzle each with 1/2 teaspoon canola oil. Bake uncovered 30 minutes or until zucchini shells are tender and golden.

Calories 100
    Calories from fat 35
Total fat 4.0 g
    Saturated fat 0.3 g
    Trans fat 0.0 g

Cholesterol 0 mg
Sodium 325 mg
Total carbohydrate 14 g
    Dietary fiber 2 g
    Sugars 4 g
Protein 3 g

EXCHANGES PER SERVING
1/2 starch
1 vegetable
1 fat

Flavorful tip A dish does not have to be smothered in canola oil to achieve golden-brown results. Just a small drizzle does the job beautifully.

Onions are used as a base for a variety of recipes, but it's their time to shine in this sweet and savory side dish.

Canola oil cooking spray

2 medium onions, peeled, trimmed, and halved crosswise

12 whole cloves

1 tablespoon light soy sauce

1 tablespoon canola oil

1 tablespoon molasses

1½ teaspoons balsamic vinegar

¼ teaspoon coarsely ground black pepper

½ teaspoon sugar

⅛ teaspoon salt

1 Preheat oven to 450°F. Coat a foil-lined baking sheet with cooking spray. Arrange the onion halves on the baking sheet and pierce evenly with the cloves.

2 Combine soy sauce, canola oil, molasses, vinegar, and black pepper in a small jar, secure with lid, and shake vigorously until completely blended. Brush 1 tablespoon of the soy mixture evenly over the onions. Bake 25 minutes, brush another tablespoon of the soy mixture evenly over the onions, and bake 5–10 minutes or until richly browned on edges and onions are tender.

3 Remove from oven and, using a flat spatula, remove the onions and place on serving platter. Spoon remaining soy mixture evenly over the onions and sprinkle evenly with the sugar and salt.

Calories 80
  Calories from fat 30
Total fat 3.5 g
  Saturated fat 0.3 g
  Trans fat 0.0 g

Cholesterol 0 mg
Sodium 225 mg
Total carbohydrate 12 g
  Dietary fiber 1 g
  Sugars 7 g
Protein 1 g

EXCHANGES PER SERVING
½ carbohydrate
1 vegetable
½ fat

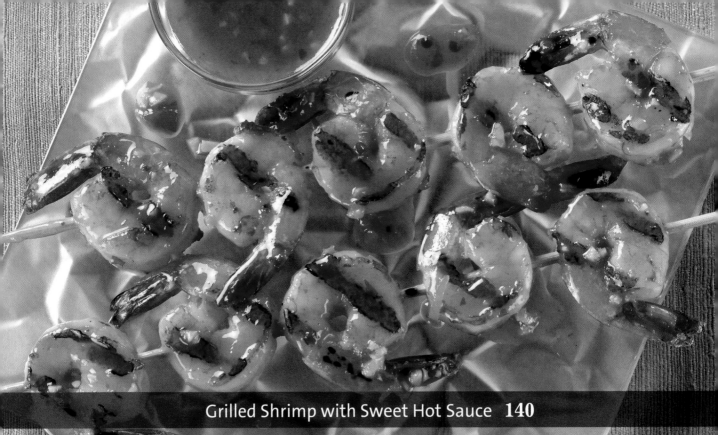

Grilled Shrimp with Sweet Hot Sauce **140**

SEAFOOD

Deviled Crab Cakes with Spicy Sauce | **138**

Scallops with Parmesan Pasta | **139**

Grilled Shrimp with Sweet Hot Sauce | **140**

Tuna Kabobs with Mild Wasabi Cream | **141**

Classic Tuna Casserole | **142**

Lime-Infused Halibut with Ginger Relish | **143**

Roasted Salmon with Adobo Cream Sauce | **144**

Sweet Tomato Creole Tilapia | **145**

Fish Tacos with Avocado Salsa | **146**

POULTRY

Baked Chicken Legs with Creamy Honey-Mustard Dip | **148**

Provençal Chicken with White Wine, Garlic, and Apricots | **149**

Grill Pan Chicken with Fiery Mango-Ginger Salsa | **151**

Chicken with Roasted Red Pepper Sauce | **152**

Panko-Parmesan Chicken with Capers | **153**

Sweet Spice-Rubbed Chicken | **154**

Chicken and Artichokes with Pasta | **155**

Jambalaya with Smoked Turkey Sausage and Chicken | **156**

Roasted Turkey with Rosemary and Sage | **158**

Hometown Turkey Meatloaf | **159**

Skillet Turkey Ham with Curried Apples and Onions | **160**

PORK

Thyme-Roasted Pork Loin with Peach-Raspberry Sauce | **161**

ENTRÉES

Pork Tenderloin, Potatoes, and Horseradish-Mustard Seed Sauce | **163**

Pork Tenderloin with Sweet Soy Marinade | **164**

Pork Medallions with Rich Onion Sauce | **165**

Hoisin Orange Pork on Asian Vegetables | **166**

Shredded Cajun Pork and Grits | **168**

Slow Cooker Smoky Pork Buns | **169**

Rosemary Pork Chops with Tomato-Caper Topping | **170**

BEEF

Grilled Flank Steak with Balsamic Vinegar and Red Wine | **171**

Coffee-Crusted Sirloin Steak | **172**

Central American-Style Beef | **173**

Beef Tenderloin and Portobellos with Marsala Sauce | **175**

Red Wine-Braised Beef with Vegetables | **176**

Drunken Beef Goulash | **177**

Creamy Beef, Mushrooms, and Noodles | **178**

Layered Mexican Casserole | **180**

MEATLESS

Barley, White Bean, and Artichoke Toss | **181**

Black Bean Burgers with Avocado-Lime Mayonnaise | **183**

Black Bean Skillet with Butternut Squash | **184**

Sweet Home Chili on Spaghetti Squash | **185**

Vegetable Pasta with Tapenade and Pine Nuts | **186**

Curried Sweet Potato and Peanut Stew | **188**

Toasted Pecan Quinoa with Red Peppers | **190**

Sesame Thai Toss with Peanut Lime Sauce | **191**

DEVILED CRAB CAKES WITH SPICY SAUCE

YIELD 4 servings | **SERVING SIZE** 1 crab cake

These crab cakes capture the true essence of the Gulf Coast.

CRAB CAKES

- ½ lb fresh crabmeat, shell pieces removed
- ¼ lb cooked shrimp, finely chopped
- ¼ cup panko bread crumbs
- 1 tablespoon canola mayonnaise
- 2 large egg whites
- ½ cup finely chopped green bell pepper
- 1 teaspoon seafood seasoning
- 1 tablespoon canola oil

SAUCE

- ⅓ cup fat-free sour cream
- 1 tablespoon canola mayonnaise
- 1 teaspoon Louisiana-style hot sauce
- ½ medium clove garlic, minced
- ⅛ teaspoon salt

- 4 lemon wedges

1 Gently mix crab cake ingredients, except canola oil, in a large bowl. Let stand 10 minutes.

2 Heat canola oil in a large nonstick skillet over medium-high heat. Immediately reduce heat to medium. Spoon crab mixture into skillet in four mounds. Flatten with the back of a spoon, creating 4-inch diameter patties, and cook 2 minutes on each side or until golden.

3 Stir together sauce ingredients in a small bowl. Serve crab cakes with sauce and lemon wedges.

Calories 165
Calories from fat 65
Total fat 7.0 g
  Saturated fat 0.5 g
  Trans fat 0.0 g

Cholesterol 90 mg
Sodium 520 mg
Total carbohydrate 5 g
  Dietary fiber 0 g
  Sugars 2 g
Protein 18 g

EXCHANGES PER SERVING
½ carbohydrate
3 lean meat

Flavorful tip Combining the canola mayonnaise with egg whites helps bind the other ingredients together, while providing moisture and flavor.

SCALLOPS WITH PARMESAN PASTA

YIELD 4 servings | **SERVING SIZE** 1 cup

Scallops add sophistication to this pasta and showcase layers of Mediterranean flavor.

¼ of 13.25-ounce package dry whole-grain spaghetti, broken in half

2 tablespoons canola oil, divided

1 lb sea scallops, rinsed and patted dry

⅛ teaspoon salt

Dash paprika

2–3 medium cloves garlic, minced

2 tablespoons white wine or water

3 tablespoons chopped fresh basil leaves, divided

2 tablespoons capers, drained

½ teaspoon black pepper

¼ cup (1 ounce) grated Parmesan cheese

1 medium plum tomato, diced

4 lemon wedges

1 Cook pasta according to package directions, omitting any salt and fat.

2 Meanwhile, heat 2 teaspoons canola oil over medium-high heat in a large nonstick skillet. Season scallops with salt and paprika and cook 2½ minutes on each side or until opaque. Place on a separate plate and cover to keep warm.

3 Reduce heat to medium, add remaining 1 tablespoon plus 1 teaspoon canola oil to skillet, add garlic, and cook 30 seconds, stirring constantly. Immediately add drained pasta, wine, 2 tablespoons basil, capers, and black pepper. Toss gently, yet thoroughly, to blend and heat through. Remove from heat, place on a serving platter, and top with Parmesan, tomato, and scallops. Sprinkle with remaining 1 tablespoon basil. Serve with lemon wedges.

Flavorful tip The secret to cooking scallops successfully is to pat them dry with paper towels before adding them to the skillet and to not overcook them. Similarly, be careful not to brown the garlic in the canola oil.

Calories 300	Cholesterol 50 mg
Calories from fat 100	Sodium 475 mg
Total fat 11.0 g	Total carbohydrate 22 g
Saturated fat 1.7 g	Dietary fiber 4 g
Trans fat 0.0 g	Sugars 1 g
	Protein 27 g

EXCHANGES PER SERVING
1½ starch
3 lean meat
1 fat

GRILLED SHRIMP WITH SWEET HOT SAUCE

YIELD 4 servings | **SERVING SIZE** 2 skewers

The orange zest brings out deep, sweet flavors in the sauce. The shrimp may be small, but they are large in taste!

1 lb raw shrimp, peeled and deveined

8 bamboo or metal skewers (10 inches long)

MARINADE

1 teaspoon chili sauce with garlic

1 tablespoon sugar

2 teaspoons cider vinegar

2 teaspoons canola oil

1 tablespoon orange juice

SAUCE

$2/3$ cup orange juice

$1/4$ cup sugar

2 tablespoons rice vinegar

1 tablespoon canola oil

1 teaspoon chili sauce with garlic

$1/2$ teaspoon salt

1 teaspoon orange zest

2 teaspoons grated fresh ginger

Canola oil cooking spray

1 Combine marinade ingredients in a small bowl and set aside. Thread shrimp on eight 10-inch metal or bamboo skewers in "C" fashion. Brush with marinade and let stand 15 minutes in the refrigerator.

2 Meanwhile, combine sauce ingredients, except zest and ginger, in a small saucepan. Bring to a boil over high heat and boil 3–4 minutes or until reduced to $1/2$ cup. Remove from heat and let cool. Add zest and ginger.

3 Coat a grill pan with cooking spray and place over high heat until hot. Remove shrimp from marinade; discard marinade. Cook shrimp 2 minutes on each side or until opaque in the center. Remove from heat. Brush sauce on shrimp or serve alongside as light dip.

Calories 255
Calories from fat 65
Total fat 7.0 g
  Saturated fat 0.7 g
  Trans fat 0.0 g

Cholesterol 185 mg
Sodium 640 mg
Total carbohydrate 21 g
  Dietary fiber 0 g
  Sugars 21 g
Protein 25 g

EXCHANGES PER SERVING
$1\frac{1}{2}$ carbohydrate
3 lean meat

Flavorful tip The sauce also goes well with grilled pork, chicken breasts, or fish fillets.

TUNA KABOBS WITH MILD WASABI CREAM

YIELD 4 servings | **SERVING SIZE** 2 skewers

These kabobs are unique and sure to please even non-seafood lovers. Wasabi can be mild to wild, but you can control the heat in this dish.

MARINADE

¼ cup reduced-sodium soy sauce
2 tablespoons fresh lime juice
1 tablespoon plus 1 teaspoon white vinegar
¼ cup minced green onions (white parts only)
4 medium cloves garlic, minced
2 tablespoons canola oil

KABOBS

4 tuna fillets (4 ounces each), rinsed, patted dry, and cut into 1-inch cubes (32 pieces total)
24 grape tomatoes
4 green onions, trimmed and each cut into 6 pieces
1 large yellow bell pepper, cut into 24 pieces
8 bamboo or metal skewers (10 inches long)
Canola oil cooking spray

CREAM SAUCE

1 tablespoon water
1 teaspoon wasabi powder
½ cup fat-free sour cream
1 teaspoon canola oil
¼ teaspoon salt

1 Stir together marinade ingredients in a shallow bowl. Set aside ¼ cup marinade for basting kabobs. Add tuna to remaining marinade and stir gently to coat. Marinate in refrigerator 30 minutes (no longer), stirring occasionally.

2 Meanwhile, prepare the cream sauce in a small bowl. Stir together water and wasabi powder until smooth, then stir in remaining sauce ingredients. Refrigerate until time of serving.

3 Remove tuna from marinade and discard marinade. Thread each skewer by alternating fish, tomato, green onions, and pepper. Each skewer will have four pieces of fish, three tomatoes, three pieces of green onion (fold green parts in half before skewering), and three pieces of pepper. Coat grill pan with cooking spray and place over high heat until hot. Brush one side of kabobs with half of reserved marinade. Add to grill pan, brushed side down, and cook 2 minutes. Brush with remaining marinade, turn, and cook 2 minutes. Do not overcook. Serve with cream sauce on the side for dipping.

Fresh tip No marinade should be left after basting the kabobs. If so, discard it to prevent cross-contamination.

			EXCHANGES PER SERVING
Calories 300	Cholesterol 45 mg		2 vegetable
Calories from fat 125	Sodium 785 mg		4 lean meat
Total fat 14.0 g	Total carbohydrate 11 g		1½ fat
Saturated fat 2.0 g	Dietary fiber 2 g		
Trans fat 0.0 g	Sugars 5 g		
	Protein 31 g		

CLASSIC TUNA CASSEROLE

YIELD 4 servings │ **SERVING SIZE** 1¼ cup

Reel in more fiber and unique seasonings with this updated comfort food. Children will take the bait and eat fish without complaint.

Canola oil cooking spray

1½ cups dry whole-grain rotini

½ cup matchstick carrots or ½ red bell pepper, thinly sliced and cut into 2-inch-long strips

½ cup frozen green peas, thawed

1 pouch (2.6 ounces) vacuum-sealed chunk light tuna, flaked

½ cup finely chopped whole green onions, divided

1 can (10.75 ounces) 98% fat-free cream of chicken or mushroom soup

⅓ cup canola mayonnaise

1 tablespoon fresh lemon juice

½ teaspoon curry powder

⅛ teaspoon salt

½ cup panko bread crumbs

1 Preheat oven to 350°F. Spray an 11 × 7-inch glass baking pan with cooking spray.

2 Cook pasta according to package directions, adding carrots or bell pepper during last 3 minutes of cooking. Drain well; place in the prepared baking pan. Top with peas and tuna, sprinkled evenly over all, and ⅓ cup green onions.

3 Stir together soup, canola mayonnaise, lemon juice, curry powder, and salt in a medium bowl. Spread over onions in baking dish. Top with bread crumbs and spray with cooking spray. Bake, uncovered, 30 minutes or until bubbly. Sprinkle with remaining green onions.

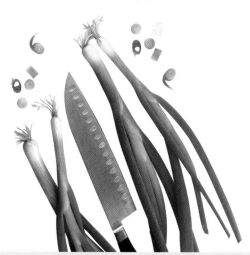

Calories 285	Cholesterol 15 mg
Calories from fat 80	Sodium 760 mg
Total fat 9.0 g	Total carbohydrate 40 g
Saturated fat 0.9 g	Dietary fiber 6 g
Trans fat 0.0 g	Sugars 4 g
	Protein 12 g

EXCHANGES PER SERVING

2½ starch
1 lean meat
1 fat

LIME-INFUSED HALIBUT
with Ginger Relish

YIELD 4 servings | **SERVING SIZE** 1 fillet

As a meaty fish, halibut stands up well to the sweet and spicy topping. This dish is perfect for a dinner party. Your guests will relish the flavors!

FISH

- 4 halibut fillets (4 ounces each), rinsed and patted dry
- 1 tablespoon fresh lime juice
- 2 teaspoons canola oil
- ½ teaspoon coarsely ground black pepper
- ¼ teaspoon salt

RELISH

- ½ cup chopped pickled ginger
- 1 medium jalapeño, seeded and finely chopped
- 2 tablespoons chopped fresh cilantro leaves
- 1 tablespoon finely chopped red onion
- 1 teaspoon canola oil
- ½ teaspoon lime zest
- 1 tablespoon fresh lime juice

  Canola oil cooking spray
- 1 lime, cut into 4 wedges (optional)

1 Place fish fillets in a 13 × 9-inch glass baking pan. Whisk together 1 tablespoon lime juice, 2 teaspoons canola oil, black pepper, and salt in a small bowl. Spoon evenly over fish and turn several times to coat evenly. Let stand 20 minutes in the refrigerator.

2 Meanwhile, combine relish ingredients in another small bowl.

3 Coat a grill pan with cooking spray; place over medium-high heat until hot. Remove fish from marinade, place on grill, and brush with any remaining marinade. Cook 5 minutes on each side or until opaque in the center and easily flaked with a fork. Place on a serving platter and squeeze lime wedges over all. Top with relish.

Flavorful tip For variation, serve the ginger relish on salmon, tuna, or mahi mahi fillets. The assertive flavors of the relish also balance nicely with grilled items, such as chicken or pork.

Calories 160
  Calories from fat 55
Total fat 6.0 g
  Saturated fat 0.6 g
  Trans fat 0.0 g

Cholesterol 35 mg
Sodium 360 mg
Total carbohydrate 2 g
  Dietary fiber 0 g
  Sugars 1 g
Protein 24 g

EXCHANGES PER SERVING
3 lean meat

ROASTED SALMON WITH ADOBO CREAM SAUCE

YIELD 4 servings | **SERVING SIZE** 1 fish fillet

Health professionals recommend consuming omega-3 fatty acids because they may protect the heart. Salmon and canola oil are both good sources of omega-3s, making this dish a heart-smart choice.

FISH
Canola oil cooking spray

4 salmon fillets (4 ounces each), rinsed and patted dry

2 teaspoons canola oil

1/2 teaspoon chili powder

1/2 teaspoon dried oregano leaves

1/4 teaspoon salt

1/4 teaspoon coarsely ground black pepper

2 tablespoons chopped fresh cilantro leaves or green onions

4 lime wedges (optional)

SAUCE
2 tablespoons canola mayonnaise

2–3 tablespoons fat-free milk

2–3 teaspoons adobo sauce

1 Preheat oven to 350°F.

2 Line a baking sheet with foil and coat with cooking spray. Place salmon on foil and drizzle canola oil evenly over fish. Combine chili powder, oregano, salt, and black pepper in a small bowl. Sprinkle salmon evenly with chili powder mixture. Place in the oven and bake 18 minutes or until fish is opaque in the center and easily flaked with a fork.

3 Meanwhile, whisk together the sauce ingredients in another small bowl. (For thinner consistency, add 2–3 teaspoons additional milk.)

4 Serve salmon with sauce on the side and sprinkled with cilantro or green onions. Serve with lime wedges.

Calories 240
  Calories from fat 125
Total fat 14.0 g
  Saturated fat 1.9 g
  Trans fat 0.0 g

Cholesterol 75 mg
Sodium 280 mg
Total carbohydrate 2 g
  Dietary fiber 0 g
  Sugars 1 g
Protein 25 g

EXCHANGES PER SERVING
3 lean meat
2 fat

Flavorful tip The salmon can be cooked on a cedar plank on the grill. Soak the plank in water for 1 hour before grilling.

SWEET TOMATO CREOLE TILAPIA

YIELD 4 servings | **SERVING SIZE** 1 fish fillet + 1 cup vegetables

The bed of warm, juicy grape tomatoes offers a hint of tartness and sweetness to complement the mild fish.

4 teaspoons canola oil, divided
1 cup diced onions
½ cup diced green bell pepper
½ cup thinly sliced celery
1 pint grape tomatoes, halved
2 teaspoons seafood seasoning, divided
½ teaspoon dried thyme leaves, divided
⅛ teaspoon salt
1 teaspoon cider vinegar
Canola oil cooking spray
4 tilapia fillets (4 ounces each), or other mild, lean white fish, rinsed and patted dry
1 lemon, cut into quarters (optional)
Hot pepper sauce (optional)

1 Heat 2 teaspoons canola oil in a large nonstick skillet over medium-high heat. Cook onions, pepper, and celery 4 minutes or until they begin to brown on the edges, stirring with two utensils. Reduce to medium-low heat; add tomatoes, 1 teaspoon seafood seasoning, and ¼ teaspoon thyme. Cover and cook 5 minutes or until vegetables are just tender. Remove from skillet, being careful not to break up tomatoes, and place on a serving platter. Sprinkle with salt and drizzle vinegar over all. Cover to keep warm.

2 Wipe skillet clean with damp paper towels. Increase heat to medium-high. Coat with cooking spray, add remaining 2 teaspoons canola oil, and tilt skillet to coat bottom lightly. Sprinkle both sides of fish with remaining 1 teaspoon seafood seasoning and thyme. Cook 3 minutes on each side or until opaque in the center and easily flaked with a fork. Place fish on top of vegetables; serve with lemon wedges and hot pepper sauce.

Calories 185
Calories from fat 65
Total fat 7.0 g
Saturated fat 1.4 g
Trans fat 0.0 g
Cholesterol 75 mg
Sodium 450 mg
Total carbohydrate 8 g
Dietary fiber 2 g
Sugars 4 g
Protein 24 g

EXCHANGES PER SERVING
2 vegetable
3 lean meat

FISH TACOS WITH AVOCADO SALSA

YIELD 4 servings | **SERVING SIZE** 2 tacos

Since experts recommend eating seafood at least twice a week, take a break from the standby beef taco and go fish!

¼ cup all-purpose flour, spooned into measuring cup and leveled

¼ cup cornmeal

½ teaspoon onion powder

½ teaspoon chili powder

4 fish fillets (1 lb total), such as tilapia, rinsed, patted dry, and cut into 8 strips total

2 tablespoons canola oil

¼ teaspoon salt

8 corn tortillas, warmed

½ medium avocado, peeled, pitted, and diced

½ cup fresh pico de gallo, salsa verde, or picante sauce

1 medium lime, cut into 8 wedges

1 Combine flour, cornmeal, onion powder, and chili powder in a shallow dish, such as a pie pan. Coat fish with mixture.

2 Heat canola oil in a large nonstick skillet over medium-high heat. Add fish; cook 3 minutes on each side or until browned and fish flakes with a fork. Place on a serving platter and sprinkle evenly with salt.

3 Place fish in warmed tortillas and top with equal amounts of avocado and pico de gallo. Squeeze a lime wedge over each tortilla.

Calories 375
 Calories from fat 125
Total fat 14.0 g
 Saturated fat 2.2 g
 Trans fat 0.0 g

Cholesterol 75 mg
Sodium 335 mg
Total carbohydrate 37 g
 Dietary fiber 5 g
 Sugars 2 g
Protein 27 g

EXCHANGES PER SERVING
2½ starch
3 lean meat
1 fat

Flavorful tip Salsa doesn't have to be limited to Mexican fare. It can be used as a spread for sandwiches and a topping for simple cuts of meat, poultry, and fish.

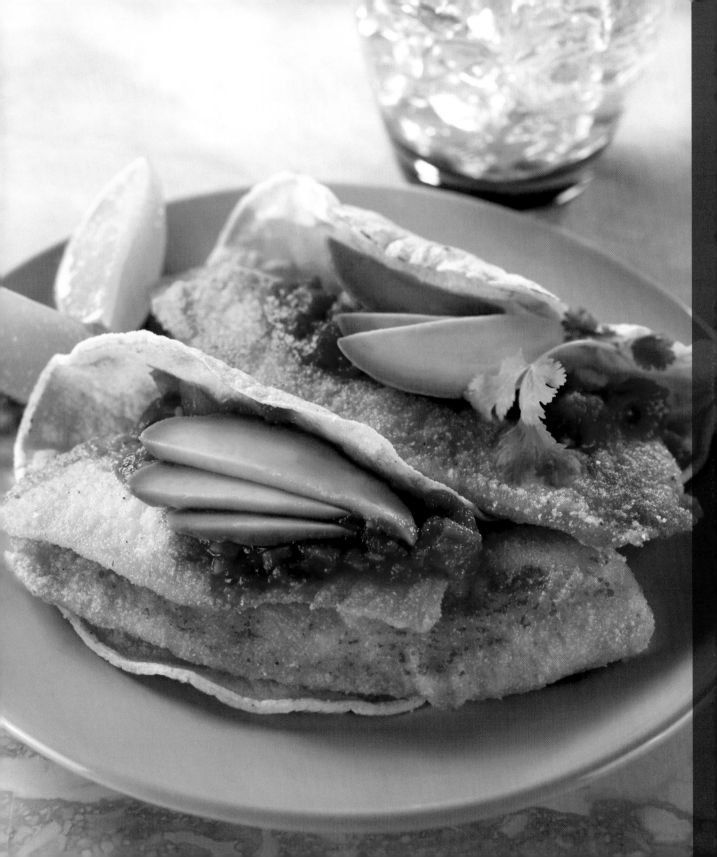

BAKED CHICKEN LEGS
with Creamy Honey-Mustard Dip

YIELD 4 servings | **SERVING SIZE** 2 drumsticks

The secret to these golden brown legs is double dipping them in buttermilk and a flour mixture prior to cooking. The delicious honey-mustard sauce will double your pleasure!

CHICKEN

- 8 chicken drumsticks, skin removed (about 2½ lbs total)
- ½ cup low-fat buttermilk
- ½ cup white whole-wheat flour, spooned into measuring cup and leveled
- 1 teaspoon paprika
- ½ teaspoon garlic powder
- ¾ teaspoon salt, divided
- 2 tablespoons canola oil
  Canola oil cooking spray

SAUCE

- 1 tablespoon honey
- 1 tablespoon yellow mustard
- 1½ tablespoons canola mayonnaise
- 1½ teaspoons fat-free milk

1 Preheat oven to 425°F. Line a baking sheet with foil and set aside.

2 Place chicken and buttermilk in a gallon-size, resealable plastic bag. Seal bag and toss back and forth to coat completely. Place flour, paprika, garlic powder, and ½ teaspoon salt in a shallow pan, such as a pie pan. Coat each piece of chicken individually and place on a dinner plate. After all have been coated with the flour mixture, repeat by placing coated chicken in buttermilk and coating again. Discard any leftover flour mixture.

3 Heat canola oil in a large nonstick skillet over medium-high heat. Add chicken and cook 3 minutes; then turn and cook an additional 3 minutes or until browned. Transfer chicken to the prepared baking sheet, discarding any remaining fat. Coat chicken with cooking spray. Bake 15 minutes, turn, and bake 15 minutes longer or until no longer pink in the center and juices run clear.

4 Meanwhile, combine sauce ingredients in a small bowl and whisk until smooth.

5 Place chicken on a serving platter and immediately sprinkle with remaining ¼ teaspoon salt. Drizzle with sauce.

		EXCHANGES PER SERVING
Calories 345	Cholesterol 120 mg	
Calories from fat 125	Sodium 525 mg	1 carbohydrate
Total fat 14.0 g	Total carbohydrate 13 g	5 lean meat
Saturated fat 2.5 g	Dietary fiber 1 g	1 fat
Trans fat 0.0 g	Sugars 6 g	
	Protein 39 g	

Fast tip To remove chicken skin easily and quickly, use two paper towels for each piece. Hold the chicken with one paper towel and pull the skin off with the other towel. The paper towels create traction to grip the skin.

PROVENÇAL CHICKEN
with White Wine, Garlic, and Apricots

YIELD 6 servings | **SERVING SIZE** 1 leg and thigh OR 1 breast + 2/3 cup vegetables

Let the heady aromas of a neighborhood bistro waft into your own home with this slow-roasted chicken in your oven.

Canola oil cooking spray

3 teaspoons canola oil, divided

4 chicken drumsticks, skin removed (about 1 lb total)

4 chicken thighs with bone in, skin removed (about 1½ lbs total)

2 chicken breasts with bone in, skin removed (about 1 lb total)

1 large onion, cut into eighths (about 6 ounces total)

1 large red bell pepper, coarsely chopped

2 medium parsnips, peeled and cut into ½-inch rounds

1 head garlic (about 12 cloves), peeled

12 dried apricot halves

1 cup reduced-sodium chicken broth

½ cup sweet white wine, such as Riesling

¾ teaspoon dried rosemary leaves

¾ teaspoon salt, divided

1 Preheat oven to 350°F. Spray a 13 × 9-inch baking dish with cooking spray.

2 Coat a large nonstick skillet with cooking spray. Add 1 teaspoon canola oil and place over medium-high heat. Add half of chicken and cook on one side 4 minutes. Transfer chicken, browned side up, to the baking dish. Repeat with cooking spray, 1 teaspoon canola oil, and remaining chicken. Transfer to baking dish.

3 Heat remaining 1 teaspoon canola oil in skillet. Add onion, pepper, parsnips, and garlic. Cook 4 minutes or until vegetables are just beginning to brown on the edges, stirring occasionally, and spoon over chicken. Add remaining ingredients, except ¼ teaspoon salt, to skillet. Bring to a boil over medium-high heat, scraping the bottom of the pan. Cook 3–4 minutes or until liquid is reduced to ¾ cup. Pour over chicken. Cover with foil and bake 55 minutes or until chicken is tender, no longer pink, and juices run clear.

4 Using a slotted spoon, place chicken and vegetables into six shallow bowls. Add ¼ teaspoon salt to broth and ladle over chicken.

Calories 355
Calories from fat 110
Total fat 12.0 g
Saturated fat 2.8 g
Trans fat 0.0 g

Cholesterol 120 mg
Sodium 495 mg
Total carbohydrate 22 g
Dietary fiber 3 g
Sugars 12 g
Protein 39 g

EXCHANGES PER SERVING
½ starch
½ fruit
1 vegetable
5 lean meat
1 fat

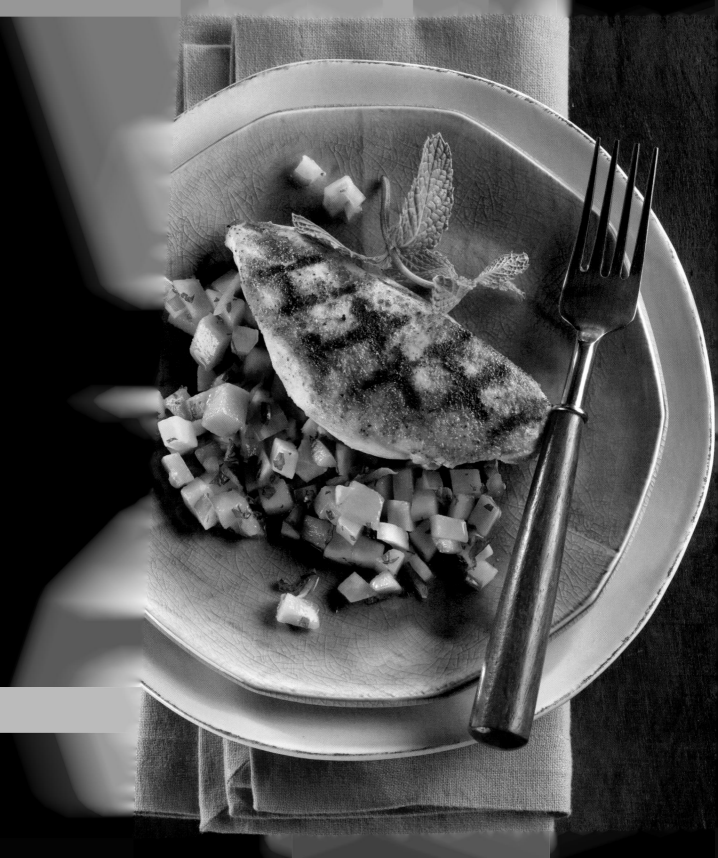

GRILL PAN CHICKEN
with Fiery Mango-Ginger Salsa

YIELD 4 servings | **SERVING SIZE** 1 chicken breast + 1/4 cup salsa

This dish offers a medley of flavors. Using salsa in place of more salt lowers the sodium content and boosts taste!

1 tablespoon canola oil

1 teaspoon curry powder

1 teaspoon sugar

1/2 teaspoon coarsely ground black pepper

1/4 teaspoon salt

4 boneless, skinless chicken breast halves (4 ounces each), rinsed, patted dry, and flattened to 1/2-inch thickness

Canola oil cooking spray

1 lemon, cut into quarters

SALSA

1 cup finely chopped mango

2–3 tablespoons chopped fresh mint leaves

1 teaspoon grated fresh ginger

2 tablespoons finely chopped red onion

1/2 teaspoon lemon zest

1 tablespoon fresh lemon juice

1 teaspoon canola oil

1 Combine 1 tablespoon canola oil, curry powder, sugar, pepper, and salt. Brush over chicken and let marinate for 15 minutes.

2 Meanwhile, stir together salsa ingredients in a small bowl.

3 Coat a grill pan with cooking spray and place over medium-high heat until hot. Add chicken, discarding any marinade. Cook chicken 4 minutes on each side or until no longer pink inside and juices run clear. Transfer to a serving platter. Squeeze lemon juice over chicken and serve with salsa.

Fast tip You can buy peeled and cut mango in a grocery store produce section to make this quick dish even faster.

Calories 205	Cholesterol 65 mg	**EXCHANGES PER SERVING**
Calories from fat 65	Sodium 175 mg	
Total fat 7.0 g	Total carbohydrate 11 g	1 fruit
Saturated fat 1.1 g	Dietary fiber 1 g	3 lean meat
Trans fat 0.0 g	Sugars 9 g	1/2 fat
	Protein 25 g	

CHICKEN WITH ROASTED RED PEPPER SAUCE

YIELD 4 servings | **SERVING SIZE** 1 chicken breast + ¼ cup sauce

This is one of the fastest sauces you'll ever make. Simply purée, heat 15 seconds, and it's ready!

Canola oil cooking spray

1 teaspoon canola oil

4 boneless, skinless chicken breast halves (4 ounces each), rinsed, patted dry, and pounded to ½-inch thickness

1 teaspoon salt-free grilling steak seasoning blend

½ teaspoon ground cumin

SAUCE

1 tablespoon canola oil

1 cup (4 ounces) roasted red peppers

1 chipotle chile pepper

¼ cup water

1 teaspoon cider vinegar

¼ cup fat-free sour cream (optional)

2 tablespoons chopped fresh cilantro leaves (optional)

1 Coat a large nonstick skillet with cooking spray. Add 1 teaspoon canola oil and heat over medium-high heat. Sprinkle chicken with seasoning blend and cumin, add chicken to skillet, and cook 4 minutes. Turn chicken. Cook 3 minutes or until no longer pink in the center and juices run clear. Remove from heat and set aside.

2 Meanwhile, combine sauce ingredients in a blender; purée until smooth.

3 Add puréed mixture to any pan residue in the skillet over medium-high heat. Stir until well blended and heated through, about 15 seconds.

4 To serve, spoon sauce onto a serving plate and arrange chicken on top. Serve with sour cream and cilantro, if desired.

Calories 175
  Calories from fat 65
Total fat 7.0 g
  Saturated fat 1.1 g
  Trans fat 0.0 g

Cholesterol 65 mg
Sodium 115 mg
Total carbohydrate 1 g
  Dietary fiber 0 g
  Sugars 1 g
Protein 24 g

EXCHANGES PER SERVING

3 lean meat
1 fat

Flavorful tip Sauces don't have to be labor-intensive. Keep the ingredients on hand to create a quick flavor-packed meal!

PANKO-PARMESAN CHICKEN WITH CAPERS

YIELD 4 servings | **SERVING SIZE** 1 chicken breast + ⅓ cup rice

Reminiscent of a restaurant-style piccata (meat sautéed in a sauce of lemon, butter, and spices), this recipe has a fraction of the fat.

- 4 boneless, skinless chicken breast halves (4 ounces each), rinsed, patted dry, and pounded to ¼-inch thickness
- 3 tablespoons fresh lemon juice, divided
- ¼ cup panko bread crumbs
- 3 tablespoons grated Parmesan cheese, divided
- 1 teaspoon paprika
- ¾ teaspoon dried oregano leaves
  Canola oil cooking spray
- 4 teaspoons canola oil, divided
- ½ cup dry white wine
- 2 medium cloves garlic, minced
- 1½–2 tablespoons capers, drained
- 1⅓ cups cooked brown rice

1 Brush both sides of chicken breasts with 1 tablespoon lemon juice.

2 Combine bread crumbs, 2 tablespoons Parmesan, paprika, and oregano in a shallow pan, such as a pie pan. Dredge each chicken breast, pressing down with your fingertips to coat with mixture, and place on a dinner plate.

3 Lightly coat a large nonstick skillet with cooking spray, add 2 teaspoons canola oil, and place over medium heat until hot. Tilt skillet to coat bottom lightly. Add two chicken breasts; cook 3 minutes on each side or until no longer pink inside and juices run clear. Transfer to a serving platter and cover to keep warm. Repeat with remaining 2 teaspoons canola oil and chicken; set aside. Increase heat to medium-high. Add remaining ingredients, except remaining Parmesan, and scrape bottom. Cook 2½–3 minutes or until mixture is reduced to ¼ cup. Spread rice evenly over four plates. Place chicken over rice, spoon sauce evenly over chicken, and sprinkle with remaining Parmesan.

Calories 295
  Calories from fat 80
Total fat 9.0 g
  Saturated fat 2.0 g
  Trans fat 0.0 g

Cholesterol 70 mg
Sodium 200 mg
Total carbohydrate 20 g
  Dietary fiber 1 g
  Sugars 1 g
Protein 28 g

EXCHANGES PER SERVING
1½ starch
3 lean meat
1 fat

SWEET SPICE-RUBBED CHICKEN

YIELD 4 servings | **SERVING SIZE** 1 chicken breast

Combining brown sugar with savory spices gives a rich, deep coloring to the chicken in this dish. Oh, and it tastes divine!

4 boneless, skinless chicken breast halves (4 ounces each), rinsed, patted dry, and pounded to ¼-inch thickness

1 tablespoon packed dark brown sugar

1 teaspoon ground coriander

½ teaspoon garlic powder

½ teaspoon black pepper

¼ teaspoon salt

¼ teaspoon ground cumin

1 tablespoon canola oil

1 teaspoon Louisiana-style hot sauce, or to taste

Canola oil cooking spray

1 lime, cut into 4 wedges (optional)

1 Place chicken on a platter. Stir together all remaining ingredients, except lime, in a small bowl. Spoon half of spice mixture on top of chicken pieces; spread evenly with the back of a spoon. Let stand 15 minutes in the refrigerator.

2 Coat a grill pan with cooking spray, and heat over medium-high heat. Add chicken, seasoned side down, and cook 4 minutes. Spoon remaining spice mixture over chicken, turn, and cook 3–4 minutes or until no longer pink in the center and juices run clear. Serve with lime wedges.

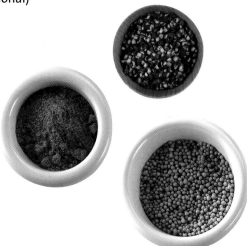

Calories 175	Cholesterol 65 mg	
Calories from fat 55	Sodium 215 mg	**EXCHANGES PER SERVING**
Total fat 6.0 g	Total carbohydrate 4 g	3 lean meat
Saturated fat 1.0 g	Dietary fiber 0 g	½ fat
Trans fat 0.0 g	Sugars 3 g	
	Protein 24 g	

Flavorful tip The canola oil ties all of the ingredients together and spreads them evenly over the chicken while keeping the spices from burning.

CHICKEN AND ARTICHOKES WITH PASTA

YIELD 4 servings | **SERVING SIZE** 1¼ cups

Combine three shades of green in this healthy pasta dish. It's so good and so good for you that it will quickly become a staple meal!

¼ of 16-ounce package dry whole-grain spaghetti noodles, broken in half

2 tablespoons canola oil, divided

¾ lb boneless, skinless chicken breasts, rinsed, patted dry, and cut into bite-size pieces

½ of 13.75-ounce can quartered artichoke hearts, drained

3 medium cloves garlic, minced

1 cup (about 1 ounce) packed baby spinach

½ cup chopped fresh basil leaves

¼ teaspoon salt

¼ cup (1 ounce) grated Parmesan cheese

1 Cook pasta according to package directions, omitting any salt or fat.

2 Meanwhile, heat 1 teaspoon canola oil in a large nonstick skillet over medium heat, tilting to coat bottom. Add chicken and cook 4 minutes or until slightly browned, stirring frequently. Add artichokes and cook, stirring constantly, 2 minutes or until chicken is no longer pink in the center and juices run clear. Transfer to a plate and set aside.

3 Add remaining canola oil and garlic to skillet and cook 15 seconds over medium heat. Remove from heat; add drained pasta, chicken mixture, spinach, basil, and salt. Toss gently, yet thoroughly, to blend. Sprinkle with Parmesan.

Fresh tip Adding the spinach leaves and basil at the very end allows the leaves to wilt slightly while retaining their vibrant color and flavor.

Calories 310
  Calories from fat 110
Total fat 12.0 g
  Saturated fat 2.2 g
  Trans fat 0.0 g

Cholesterol 55 mg
Sodium 370 mg
Total carbohydrate 24 g
  Dietary fiber 4 g
  Sugars 1 g
Protein 26 g

EXCHANGES PER SERVING
1½ starch
1 vegetable
3 lean meat
1 fat

JAMBALAYA
with Smoked Turkey Sausage and Chicken
YIELD 4 servings | **SERVING SIZE** 1⅓ cups

Jambalaya is a Creole dish of Spanish and French influence. Turmeric gives this version a brilliant yellow hue.

2 tablespoons canola oil, divided

1½ cups smoked turkey sausage, thinly sliced

¼ lb boneless, skinless chicken breast, cut into bite-size pieces

1 cup chopped red bell pepper

1 cup chopped green bell pepper

½ cup chopped onion

1 medium celery stalk, thinly sliced

1¼ cups water

¾ cup quick-cooking brown rice

½ lb peeled, deveined raw shrimp

2 dried bay leaves

½ teaspoon dried thyme leaves

⅛ teaspoon ground turmeric (optional)

2–3 teaspoons Louisiana-style hot sauce

½ teaspoon salt

1 Heat 1 teaspoon canola oil in a large nonstick skillet over medium-high heat. Add sausage and cook 3 minutes. Remove from skillet and set aside.

2 In the same skillet, heat another 1 teaspoon canola oil, add chicken, and cook 2 minutes, stirring frequently, until pieces are no longer pink. Add another 1 teaspoon canola oil; cook peppers, onion, and celery 4 minutes or until onions are translucent. Add water and bring to a boil over medium-high heat. Stir in rice, shrimp, bay leaves, thyme, and turmeric. Return to a boil, reduce heat, cover tightly, and simmer 10 minutes.

3 Remove from heat. Add sausage, remaining 1 tablespoon canola oil, hot sauce, and salt. Cook uncovered 2 minutes to thicken slightly but retain moist, saucy texture. Remove bay leaves. Serve with additional hot sauce, if desired.

Calories 305
  Calories from fat 110
Total fat 12.0 g
  Saturated fat 2.4 g
  Trans fat 0.0 g

Cholesterol 130 mg
Sodium 805 mg
Total carbohydrate 23 g
  Dietary fiber 2 g
  Sugars 4 g
Protein 23 g

EXCHANGES PER SERVING
1 starch
1 vegetable
3 lean meat
1½ fat

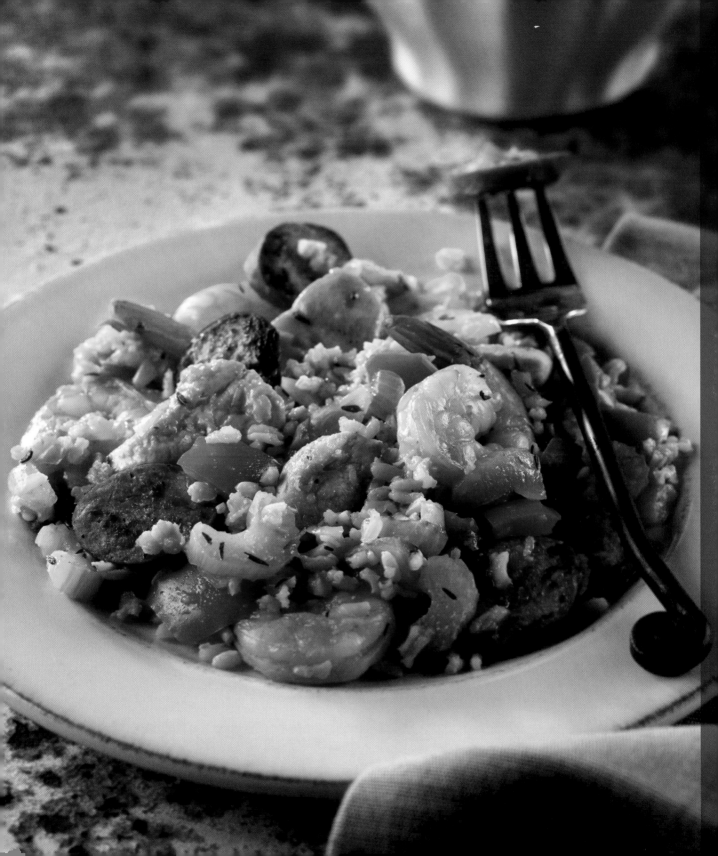

ROASTED TURKEY WITH ROSEMARY AND SAGE

YIELD 11 servings | **SERVING SIZE** 2–3 slices (3 ounces)

Don't limit turkey to just holidays. Make every day a special occasion with this savory dish!

Canola oil cooking spray

2 tablespoons canola oil

1½ teaspoons chopped fresh rosemary leaves

½ teaspoon dried sage, crumbled

¼ cup finely chopped fresh parsley leaves

2 medium cloves garlic, minced

2 teaspoons lemon zest

2 tablespoons fresh lemon juice

½ teaspoon coarsely ground black pepper

½ teaspoon salt

5 lbs turkey breast (bone-in), thawed, rinsed, and patted dry

Paprika

1 Preheat oven to 325°F. Place a roasting rack in a pan, and spray with cooking spray.

2 Combine all ingredients, except turkey and paprika, in a small bowl. Separate skin from turkey meat by gently sliding fingers between, being careful not to tear the skin if possible. Stuff parsley mixture under skin, pull skin over mixture, and sprinkle lightly with paprika over all. Place on the rack, breast side up, and roast for 1 hour 45 minutes or until a meat thermometer inserted into thickest part of breast reads 165°F. Let stand 15 minutes. Carefully remove skin and discard it, leaving parsley mixture on turkey. Thinly slice turkey and serve.

Calories 145
Calories from fat 25
Total fat 3.0 g
  Saturated fat 0.4 g
  Trans fat 0.0 g

Cholesterol 75 mg
Sodium 155 mg
Total carbohydrate 1 g
  Dietary fiber 0 g
  Sugars 0 g
Protein 27 g

EXCHANGES PER SERVING
3 lean meat

Flavorful tip Adding the canola oil under the skin helps bring out the flavors of the fresh herbs and lemon zest while keeping the turkey moist. So keep the skin on for cooking, but don't forget to discard it before serving.

HOMETOWN TURKEY MEATLOAF

YIELD 4 servings | **SERVING SIZE** 1 mini loaf

These individual meatloaves make great leftovers because they can be frozen in separate bags and used whenever a quick dinner or microwave lunch is needed.

2 tablespoons ketchup

1 can (8 ounces) tomato sauce with Italian seasonings, divided

3 teaspoons canola oil, divided

¾ lb lean ground turkey

¾ cup finely chopped green pepper

½ cup finely chopped onion

2 egg whites

1 teaspoon Worcestershire sauce

½ teaspoon dried Italian seasoning

¼ teaspoon salt

½ cup quick-cooking oats

1 Preheat oven to 350°F. Line a baking sheet with foil.

2 Combine ketchup, 2 tablespoons tomato sauce, and 1 teaspoon canola oil in a small bowl and set aside.

3 Combine remaining ingredients in a large bowl. On a baking sheet, shape turkey mixture into four individual meatloaf ovals, about 3 × 4½ inches. Bake 30 minutes or until a meat thermometer inserted into thickest part of meatloaf reads 165°F. Remove from oven. Using the back of a spoon, evenly spread the sauce over the top and sides. Let stand 5 minutes before serving.

Fresh tip Read labels when buying ground turkey because some varieties can be quite high in saturated fat. Look for the words "lean" and/or "breast meat" to find the leaner versions.

Calories 245
 Calories from fat 90
Total fat 10.0 g
 Saturated fat 2.3 g
 Trans fat 0.0 g

Cholesterol 60 mg
Sodium 630 mg
Total carbohydrate 17 g
 Dietary fiber 3 g
 Sugars 4 g
Protein 21 g

EXCHANGES PER SERVING
1 carbohydrate
3 lean meat
1 fat

SKILLET TURKEY HAM
with Curried Apples and Onions

YIELD 4 servings | **SERVING SIZE** 1 slice turkey ham + 1/3 cup topping

Enjoy these warm and wintery flavors any time of year with this very simple, comforting dish.

1½ tablespoons canola oil, divided

½ lb turkey ham, cut into 4 slices

½ cup finely chopped onion

2 small Gala apples (8 ounces total), halved, cored, and diced

3 tablespoons dried cranberries

½ teaspoon curry powder

¼ teaspoon ground cumin

1 teaspoon orange zest

1 Heat ½ tablespoon canola oil in a large nonstick skillet over medium-high heat. Tilt skillet to coat bottom lightly. Add ham; cook 3 minutes, turn, and cook 1 minute more. Transfer to a plate and cover to keep warm.

2 Add remaining 1 tablespoon canola oil to the skillet and heat. Add onion and cook 2 minutes. Add apples and cranberries and cook 4 minutes until the apples are tender crisp, stirring frequently. Stir in curry powder, cumin, and zest; remove from heat. Spoon evenly over ham slices.

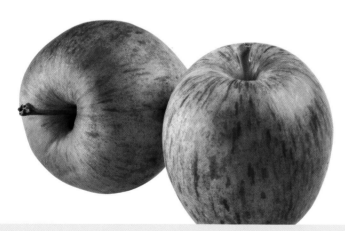

		EXCHANGES PER SERVING	
Calories 170	Cholesterol 35 mg		*Flavorful tip* Turkey "ham" is made from turkey thigh meat, which is cured and smoked. It is a lower fat alternative to pork ham.
Calories from fat 70	Sodium 505 mg	1 fruit	
Total fat 8.0 g	Total carbohydrate 15 g	1 lean meat	
Saturated fat 1.3 g	Dietary fiber 2 g	1½ fat	
Trans fat 0.0 g	Sugars 11 g		
	Protein 9 g		

THYME-ROASTED PORK LOIN
with Peach-Raspberry Sauce

YIELD 8 servings | **SERVING SIZE** about 5 slices (3 ounces) pork

Peach, raspberry, and thyme—a terrific flavor trio—go very well with pork.

Canola oil cooking spray
1 cup peach fruit spread
¼ cup balsamic vinegar
1 tablespoon Worcestershire sauce
½ teaspoon dried red pepper flakes (optional)
1 tablespoon canola oil
2½ lbs boneless, center-cut pork loin roast, trimmed of fat
1 teaspoon garlic salt
1 teaspoon dried thyme leaves, crushed
1 teaspoon coarsely ground black pepper
½ cup fresh raspberries or frozen unsweetened raspberries, thawed

1 Preheat oven to 425°F and lightly coat 13 × 9-inch baking pan with cooking spray. Combine fruit spread, vinegar, Worcestershire sauce, and pepper flakes in a small bowl; set aside.

2 Heat canola oil in a large nonstick skillet over medium-high heat. Sprinkle pork with garlic salt, thyme, and pepper. Brown meat for 5 minutes on one side; then turn and brown for 1 minute on the other side. Place pork, richly browned side up, in prepared baking pan. Bake 30 minutes.

3 To pan residue in skillet, add half of fruit spread mixture, bring to a boil over medium-high heat, and cook 15 seconds, stirring constantly. Remove from heat and place mixture in the refrigerator until needed. After pork has cooked for 30 minutes, baste it with refrigerated mixture. If fruit spread mixture is too thick, heat it in the microwave for 20 seconds or until slightly melted. Cook pork 5–10 minutes longer or until a meat thermometer inserted into thickest part of loin registers 160°F. Place on a cutting board and let stand 5 minutes before slicing.

4 Place raspberries and remaining fruit spread mixture in a medium saucepan. Bring just to a boil over medium-high heat and continue boiling 2–3 minutes or until it is reduced to ½ cup liquid. Remove from heat and spoon sauce evenly over pork.

Fast tip Leftover pork loin and sauce make great sandwiches. Try mixing a little coarse-grain Dijon mustard with the sauce for a flavorful spread. If desired, apricot fruit spread may be substituted for peach in this recipe.

Calories 300
  Calories from fat 100
Total fat 11.0 g
  Saturated fat 3.3 g
  Trans fat 0.0 g

Cholesterol 70 mg
Sodium 250 mg
Total carbohydrate 23 g
  Dietary fiber 1 g
  Sugars 18 g
Protein 27 g

EXCHANGES PER SERVING
1½ carbohydrate
3 lean meat
1 fat

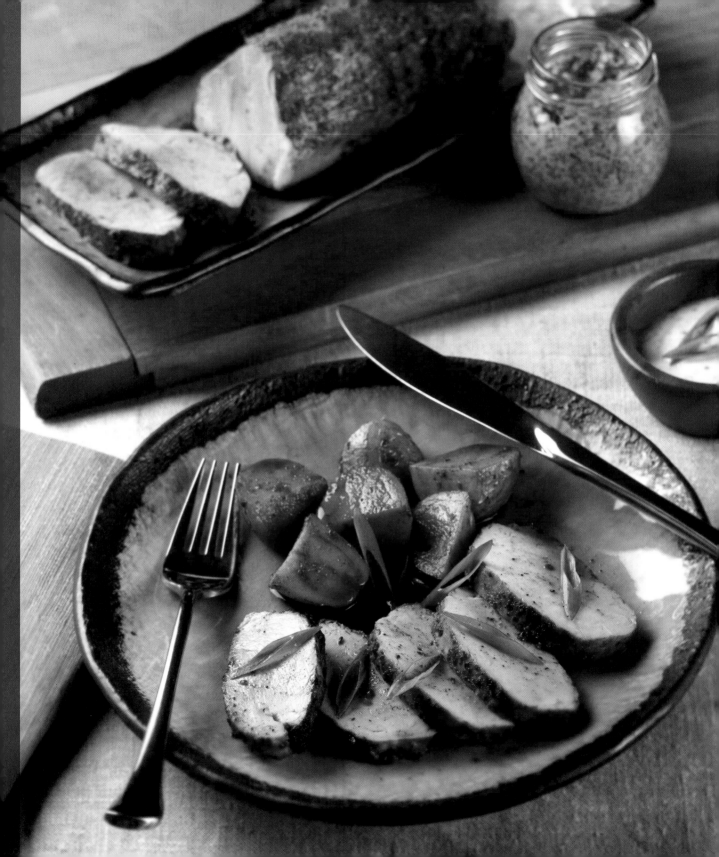

PORK TENDERLOIN, POTATOES,
and Horseradish-Mustard Seed Sauce

YIELD 4 servings | **SERVING SIZE** about 5 slices (3 ounces) pork + 5 potato wedges

The meat and potatoes in this zesty dish never tasted so good!

1 tablespoon canola oil

1 lb pork tenderloin

1 teaspoon salt-free seasoning, such as steak seasoning blend

½ teaspoon salt, divided

5 new potatoes (about 1 lb total), quartered

Paprika

SAUCE

⅓ cup fat-free sour cream

2 tablespoons canola mayonnaise

1 tablespoon water

2 teaspoons prepared horseradish

2 teaspoons coarse-grain Dijon mustard

1 Preheat oven to 425°F. Cover baking sheet with foil.

2 Heat canola oil in a large nonstick skillet over medium-high heat. Sprinkle pork tenderloin with seasoning blend and ¼ teaspoon salt. Cook 3 minutes, turn, and cook 2 more minutes. Place pork on the prepared baking sheet.

3 Add potatoes to skillet and sprinkle with paprika. Toss to coat, preferably with a heat-resistant rubber spatula, and cook for 1 minute. Place potatoes around pork and roast for 18–20 minutes or until a meat thermometer inserted into thickest part of meat registers 160°F.

4 Meanwhile, combine sauce ingredients in a small bowl.

5 Place pork on a cutting board and let stand 5 minutes before slicing. Pull sides of foil up around potatoes, seal foil, and let stand. Slice pork and place on a serving platter. Sprinkle remaining ¼ teaspoon salt over potatoes and place potatoes around pork with any accumulated juices. Serve with sauce.

Flavorful tip Tossing the cut potatoes in paprika and the pan residue adds a rich brown, glistening color to the potatoes.

Calories 265
    Calories from fat 80
Total fat 9.0 g
    Saturated fat 1.3 g
    Trans fat 0.0 g

Cholesterol 65 mg
Sodium 465 mg
Total carbohydrate 19 g
    Dietary fiber 2 g
    Sugars 2 g
Protein 25 g

EXCHANGES PER SERVING
1 starch
3 lean meat
1 fat

PORK TENDERLOIN WITH SWEET SOY MARINADE

YIELD 4 servings | **SERVING SIZE** about 5 slices (3 ounces) pork

This sweet and savory marinade brings out the best in the pork. It is sure to wow dinner guests every time.

MARINADE

- 2 tablespoons packed dark brown sugar
- 3 tablespoons cider vinegar
- 3 tablespoons reduced-sodium soy sauce
- 2 tablespoons canola oil
- ½ teaspoon coarsely ground black pepper
- ¼ teaspoon dried red pepper flakes (optional)
- ½ teaspoon grated fresh ginger
- ⅛ teaspoon salt
- 1 lb pork tenderloin
  Canola oil cooking spray
- 1 tablespoon water

1 Combine marinade ingredients in a large, resealable plastic bag. Seal tightly and shake back and forth until well blended. Reserve 2 tablespoons of mixture in a separate small bowl. Add ginger and salt to reserved mixture; refrigerate. Add tenderloin to marinade in the bag, seal, toss to coat, and refrigerate overnight or for at least 8 hours, turning occasionally.

2 Preheat oven to 425°F.

3 Coat a large nonstick skillet with cooking spray and place over medium-high heat until hot. Remove pork from marinade; discard marinade. Place pork in the skillet, and cook 3 minutes; then turn and cook other side for 1 minute. Place in an 11 × 7-inch baking pan, move to oven, and bake for 12 minutes. Pour reserved 2 tablespoons soy mixture over pork and bake 3–5 minutes more or until a meat thermometer inserted into thickest part of meat registers 160°F.

4 Remove pork from pan and place on a cutting board. Let stand 10 minutes before slicing. Meanwhile, add water to pan residue, and stir, scraping the bottom and sides, preferably with a heat-resistant rubber spatula. Spoon liquid over pork while it is standing.

Calories 170
Calories from fat 55
Total fat 6.0 g
Saturated fat 1.3 g
Trans fat 0.0 g

Cholesterol 60 mg
Sodium 335 mg
Total carbohydrate 4 g
Dietary fiber 0 g
Sugars 4 g
Protein 22 g

EXCHANGES PER SERVING
3 lean meat
½ fat

Flavorful tip Canola oil is the perfect base for marinades as it lets ingredient flavors shine through and won't overpower the meat.

PORK MEDALLIONS WITH RICH ONION SAUCE

YIELD 4 servings | **SERVING SIZE** 2 slices pork

Tender, thin slices of pork tenderloin are offset by the robust taste of the sauce.

1 lb pork tenderloin, cut into 8 slices, pounded to ⅛-inch thickness

1 teaspoon salt-free grill seasoning blend

3 teaspoons canola oil, divided

1 cup thinly sliced onions

2 medium cloves garlic, minced

¾ teaspoon Dijon mustard

2 teaspoons white whole-wheat flour

½ cup water

2 teaspoons low-sodium beef bouillon granules

1 Sprinkle both sides of pork with seasoning blend.

2 Heat 1 teaspoon canola oil in a large nonstick skillet over medium-high heat. Tilt skillet to coat bottom. Add half of pork slices and cook 2 minutes; then turn and cook 1 minute or until juices run clear. Set aside on a plate. Repeat with 1 teaspoon canola oil and remaining pork and place on the plate.

3 Heat remaining 1 teaspoon canola oil, tilt skillet, and add onions. Reduce heat to medium and cook for 3 minutes or until onions are translucent. Stir in garlic. Remove skillet from heat and stir in remaining ingredients until well blended.

4 Return to heat and add pork and any accumulated juices. Turn pieces over several times to coat with onion mixture, reduce to medium-low heat, cover tightly, and simmer 10 minutes or until pork is very tender and juices run clear.

Fresh tip To thinly pound pork, place an 18-inch sheet of plastic wrap on the counter and lay pork on top. Top with a sheet of plastic wrap. Use a meat pounder, mallet, or the side of a can to pound the pork to ⅛ inch or more. Thinness is the key to tenderness.

Calories 170	Cholesterol 60 mg
Calories from fat 55	Sodium 515 mg
Total fat 6.0 g	Total carbohydrate 5 g
Saturated fat 1.3 g	Dietary fiber 1 g
Trans fat 0.0 g	Sugars 2 g
	Protein 23 g

EXCHANGES PER SERVING
1 vegetable
3 lean meat

HOISIN ORANGE PORK ON ASIAN VEGETABLES

YIELD 4 servings | **SERVING SIZE** about 1¼ cups

Hoisin is a sweet and spicy sauce widely used in Chinese cooking that complements pork extremely well. It's a mixture of soybeans, garlic, chile peppers, and various spices.

¾ lb boneless pork chops, trimmed of fat, cut into very thin strips

1 tablespoon reduced-sodium soy sauce

3 tablespoons unsalted, dry-roasted peanuts, toasted and finely chopped

2 medium carrots, thinly sliced diagonally

2 cups small broccoli florets

1 medium onion, cut into ¼-inch wedges

¼ cup water

1 tablespoon plus 1 teaspoon canola oil, divided

SAUCE

3 tablespoons hoisin sauce

2 tablespoons cider vinegar

1 tablespoon sugar

2 teaspoons orange zest

¼ teaspoon dried red pepper flakes

1 Place pork strips on a dinner plate, spoon 1 tablespoon soy sauce over all, and toss to coat well. Let stand 15 minutes in the refrigerator.

2 Meanwhile, heat a large nonstick skillet over medium-high heat. Add nuts and cook 2–3 minutes or until they begin to brown, stirring frequently. Place on a separate plate and set aside.

3 Place carrots, broccoli, onion, and water in a microwave-safe shallow pan, such as a glass pie pan, cover, and microwave on high 2 minutes or until vegetables are just tender crisp. Drain in a colander, shaking off any excess liquid.

4 Combine sauce ingredients in a small bowl; set aside. Heat 1 teaspoon canola oil in a large nonstick skillet over medium-high heat. Tilt skillet to coat lightly, add pork, and cook 3 minutes or until lightly pink in the center and juices run clear, using two utensils to toss easily. Set aside on a separate plate.

5 Heat remaining 1 tablespoon canola oil, add vegetables, and cook 4 minutes or until tender crisp and beginning to lightly brown on the edges. Place vegetables on a serving platter. Add pork and any accumulated juices to skillet, cook 30 seconds to heat thoroughly, and place on top of vegetables on serving platter. Add sauce to skillet and cook 20–30 seconds to heat, stirring constantly, until reduced slightly. Spoon over pork and sprinkle with nuts. Serve immediately.

		EXCHANGES PER SERVING	
Calories 275	Cholesterol 45 mg		*Fast tip* Stir-fries cook quickly, so it's critical to have everything prepped before starting to cook. Hoisin sauce is found in the Asian section of major supermarkets.
Calories from fat 125	Sodium 370 mg	½ carbohydrate	
Total fat 14.0 g	Total carbohydrate 17 g	2 vegetable	
Saturated fat 2.9 g	Dietary fiber 3 g	2 lean meat	
Trans fat 0.0 g	Sugars 11 g	2 fat	
	Protein 20 g		

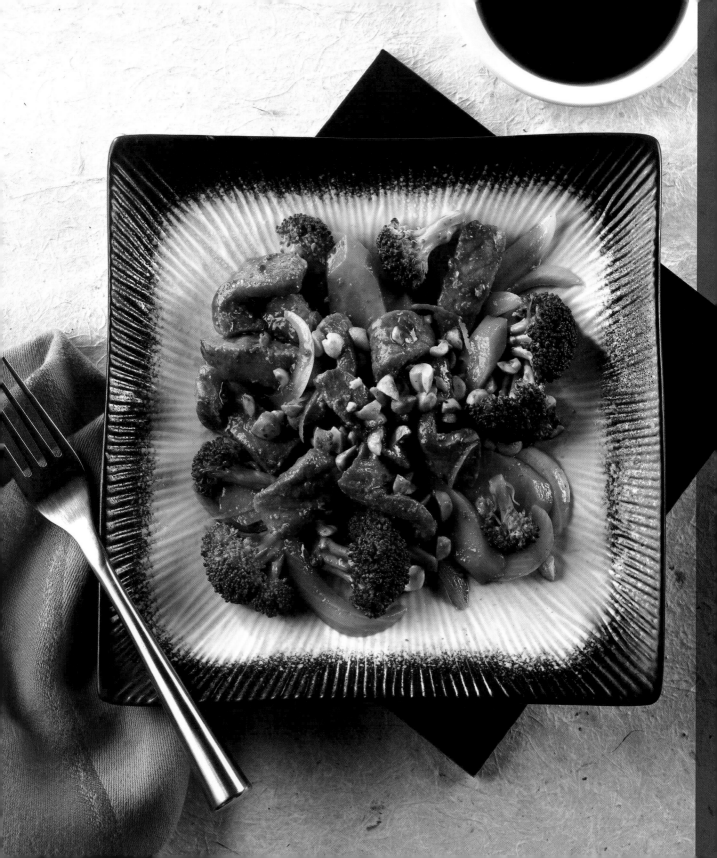

SHREDDED CAJUN PORK AND GRITS

YIELD 4 servings | **SERVING SIZE** ¾ cup pork mixture + ½ cup grits

Browning flour in canola oil in this recipe creates a roux, which is traditionally made with butter or bacon grease. This healthier, full-flavored roux is fantastic over grits and spicy pork.

Canola oil cooking spray
2 tablespoons canola oil
1 lb boneless pork chops
2 tablespoons all-purpose flour
1 cup chopped onions
1 cup chopped green pepper
1 medium celery stalk, sliced
1 can (14.5 ounces) stewed Cajun tomatoes
½ teaspoon dried thyme leaves
2 dried bay leaves
½ cup dry quick-cooking grits

1 Spray a 3½- to 4-quart slow cooker with cooking spray.

2 Coat a medium nonstick skillet with cooking spray and place over medium-high heat until hot. Add pork and cook 2 minutes to brown; turn and cook 2 minutes.

3 Place pork in the slow cooker. Add canola oil to pan residue in the skillet. Sprinkle flour evenly over the bottom of the skillet and cook 5 minutes until richly browned, stirring constantly (preferably with a heat-proof spatula). Add onions, pepper, and celery, and toss to coat. Add tomatoes, thyme, and bay leaves. Stir until well blended. Pour over pork. Cover tightly and cook on high setting for 4 hours or low setting for 8 hours, until a meat thermometer reads 160°F.

4 Shred pork and return to slow cooker. Remove bay leaves. Stir to blend. Cook grits according to package directions, omitting any salt or fat. Serve pork mixture over grits.

Calories 355
  Calories from fat 135
Total fat 15.0 g
  Saturated fat 3.5 g
  Trans fat 0.0 g

Cholesterol 50 mg
Sodium 275 mg
Total carbohydrate 31 g
  Dietary fiber 4 g
  Sugars 7 g
Protein 24 g

EXCHANGES PER SERVING
1 starch
3 vegetable
2 lean meat
2½ fat

SLOW COOKER SMOKY PORK BUNS

YIELD 8 servings | **SERVING SIZE** 1/3 cup mixture + 1 bun

Nothing tastes more like barbeque than these sandwiches...without the grill!

Canola oil cooking spray
6 teaspoons canola oil, divided
4 bone-in pork chops, trimmed of fat (about 1 1/2 lbs total)
1 1/2 cups diced onions
1/4 cup water
1/4 cup mild picante sauce
1/2 cup hickory smoked barbeque sauce, divided
2 tablespoons cider vinegar
1 teaspoon Worcestershire sauce
1/2 teaspoon ground cumin
8 whole-wheat hamburger buns, split, toasted

1 Spray a 3 1/2- or 4-quart slow cooker with cooking spray.

2 Heat 1 teaspoon canola oil in a large nonstick skillet over medium-high heat. Tilt skillet to coat bottom lightly. Add pork chops and cook 4 minutes on one side. Place pork, browned side up, in the slow cooker.

3 Add 2 teaspoons canola oil to pan residue, tilting skillet to coat bottom. Add onions and cook 8–9 minutes or until richly browned, stirring frequently. Add 1/4 cup water to onions and stir until well blended, scraping bottom. Remove from heat. Stir in picante sauce and 2 tablespoons barbeque sauce. Place over pork. Cover and cook on high setting for 3 hours or low setting for 6 hours until a meat thermometer reads 160°F.

4 Remove meat and shred with a fork, discarding any bones. Return to slow cooker and add remaining ingredients, except buns. To serve, spoon equal amounts of pork mixture on buns.

Flavorful tip Adding some ingredients at the end of the cooking time allows the sauce flavors to be more pronounced. Cool any leftovers and place individual servings in small freezer bags to have on hand for a quick pre-portioned meal.

Calories 270	Cholesterol 35 mg
Calories from fat 80	Sodium 480 mg
Total fat 9.0 g	Total carbohydrate 31 g
Saturated fat 1.9 g	Dietary fiber 4 g
Trans fat 0.0 g	Sugars 9 g
	Protein 17 g

EXCHANGES PER SERVING
2 starch
2 lean meat
1/2 fat

ROSEMARY PORK CHOPS
with Tomato-Caper Topping

YIELD 4 servings | **SERVING SIZE** 1 pork chop

The assertive flavor of rosemary makes this dish, but it's supported by wine, capers, and sweet grape tomatoes, which all dazzle the taste buds.

1 tablespoon canola oil

4 boneless pork chops (4 ounces each)

¾ teaspoon chopped fresh rosemary leaves, divided

1 large shallot, sliced (1 ounce)

1 pint grape tomatoes, halved

2 tablespoons capers, drained

¼ cup dry white wine, such as chardonnay

¼ teaspoon salt

1 Heat canola oil in a large nonstick skillet over medium-high heat. Sprinkle one side of pork chops with ½ teaspoon rosemary and cook, seasoned side down, 4 minutes. Turn pork, sprinkle shallot around meat, and cook 4 more minutes or until juices run clear. Transfer pork to a platter.

2 To pan residue, add remaining ingredients, except remaining rosemary, and cook, stirring constantly, for 2 minutes or until tomatoes are just beginning to wilt. Spoon evenly over pork chops and sprinkle with remaining ¼ teaspoon rosemary.

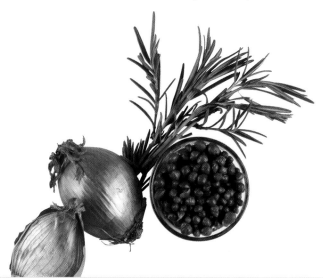

Calories 200
Calories from fat 100
Total fat 11.0 g
　Saturated fat 3.1 g
　Trans fat 0.0 g

Cholesterol 45 mg
Sodium 310 mg
Total carbohydrate 3 g
　Dietary fiber 1 g
　Sugars 1 g
Protein 19 g

EXCHANGES PER SERVING
3 lean meat
1½ fat

Flavorful tip Serve this dish on top of 2 cups cooked (4 ounces dry) whole-grain spaghetti to catch the juices as they trickle down from the chop!

GRILLED FLANK STEAK
with Balsamic Vinegar and Red Wine

YIELD 4 servings | **SERVING SIZE** 3–4 slices (3 ounces) beef

Canola oil in this balsamic-wine marinade maximizes moisture in the meat.

MARINADE

- 2 tablespoons canola oil
- 1 teaspoon dried oregano leaves
- ½ cup dry red wine
- ¼ cup balsamic vinegar
- 2 tablespoons Worcestershire sauce
- 2 medium cloves garlic, minced
- 1 teaspoon coarsely ground black pepper

- 1 lb flank steak
- Canola oil cooking spray
- 1½ teaspoons sugar
- ¼ teaspoon salt

1 Combine all marinade ingredients in a large, resealable bag, seal tightly, and shake back and forth until well blended. Pour ¼ cup of marinade in a separate container and set aside. Add beef to remaining marinade in the resealable bag. Seal and gently turn back and forth to coat. Refrigerate for 24–48 hours, turning occasionally. Refrigerate reserved marinade as well.

2 Remove meat from bag and discard marinade. Spray a grill pan with cooking spray. Place grill pan over medium-high heat until hot. Add beef and cook 4–5 minutes on each side or to desired doneness. Place meat on a cutting board and let stand 5 minutes before thinly slicing diagonally.

3 Meanwhile, place reserved marinade, sugar, and salt in a small saucepan and bring to a boil over medium-high heat. Continue boiling for 1–2 minutes or until liquid is reduced to 2 tablespoons. Spoon over steak to serve.

Flavorful tip Cutting beef across the grain allows for a more tender serving of meat.

Calories 185
Calories from fat 70
Total fat 8.0 g
Saturated fat 2.6 g
Trans fat 0.0 g

Cholesterol 40 mg
Sodium 220 mg
Total carbohydrate 4 g
Dietary fiber 0 g
Sugars 3 g
Protein 22 g

EXCHANGES PER SERVING
3 lean meat
1 fat

COFFEE-CRUSTED SIRLOIN STEAK

YIELD 4 servings | **SERVING SIZE** 1 steak

Coffee is used to intensify beef and chocolate dishes. It's great in desserts like chocolate cake, but equally as delicious in savory dishes, such as chili, stew, and even steak...as you'll quickly discover in this recipe.

- 1 lb boneless sirloin steak, about ¾-inch thick, cut into 4 pieces
- ¾ teaspoon salt-free steak seasoning
- 1 teaspoon chili powder
- 2 teaspoons instant coffee granules
- 1 tablespoon canola oil
- ¼ cup water
- 1 tablespoon balsamic vinegar
- ½ teaspoon coarsely ground black pepper
- ¼ teaspoon salt

1 Sprinkle steak evenly with steak seasoning and chili powder. Let stand 10 minutes at room temperature. Sprinkle evenly with coffee granules and press down with your fingertips to allow granules to adhere.

2 Heat canola oil in a large nonstick skillet over medium-high heat. Tilt skillet to coat bottom lightly. Cook steak 2 minutes; turn and cook 1 minute more or until desired doneness is reached. Set aside on a serving platter. Add water, vinegar, pepper, and salt to skillet. Bring to a boil over medium-high heat and cook for 1½–2 minutes or until reduced to 2 tablespoons.

Calories 170	Cholesterol 40 mg
Calories from fat 70	Sodium 200 mg
Total fat 8.0 g	Total carbohydrate 2 g
Saturated fat 1.9 g	Dietary fiber 0 g
Trans fat 0.2 g	Sugars 1 g
	Protein 22 g

EXCHANGES PER SERVING
3 lean meat
½ fat

Fast tip Sirloin is a tender cut of beef, but it can become overcooked and tough. It's best to cook sirloin quickly. Let it stand for a few minutes to continue cooking and then thinly slice the meat against the grain.

CENTRAL AMERICAN-STYLE BEEF

YIELD 4 servings | **SERVING SIZE** 1 steak

The marinade for the beef is similar to Argentinean chimichurri, a spicy sauce used with grilled meat. It is found on menus in Central America, especially Nicaragua.

1 lb boneless beef round steak, flattened to ⅛-inch thickness or thinner if possible

MARINADE

1 tablespoon canola oil

2 tablespoons fresh lime juice

¼ teaspoon salt

¼ teaspoon black pepper

TOPPING

2 tablespoons minced fresh cilantro leaves

2 tablespoons minced onion

2 tablespoons minced red bell pepper

1 tablespoon canola oil

1–1½ tablespoons white vinegar

¼ teaspoon dried oregano leaves

1 medium clove garlic, minced

⅛ teaspoon dried red pepper flakes

½ teaspoon salt

Canola oil cooking spray

1 medium lime, quartered (optional)

1 Cut beef into four pieces and place in a glass 13 × 9-inch baking pan. Combine marinade ingredients and pour over beef. Turn beef several times to coat. Cover with plastic wrap and refrigerate overnight or for at least 8 hours, turning occasionally.

2 At time of serving, combine topping ingredients in a small bowl.

3 Coat a grill pan with cooking spray and place over high heat until hot. Remove beef from marinade, discard marinade, and place 2 beef slices on the grill pan. Cook 2 minutes, turn, cook 1 more minute, and place on a serving platter. Cover to keep warm. Repeat with remaining beef slices and serve topped with cilantro mixture. Serve with lime wedges.

Flavorful tip The thinner the beef, the more flavorful. Cook the beef quickly over very high heat to impart peak flavors and texture. Also, prepare the topping as close to serving time as possible, so the flavors will be heightened, not blended.

Calories 225	Cholesterol 75 mg
Calories from fat 115	Sodium 470 mg
Total fat 13.0 g	Total carbohydrate 2 g
Saturated fat 2.5 g	Dietary fiber 0 g
Trans fat 0.2 g	Sugars 1 g
	Protein 25 g

EXCHANGES PER SERVING
3 lean meat
1½ fat

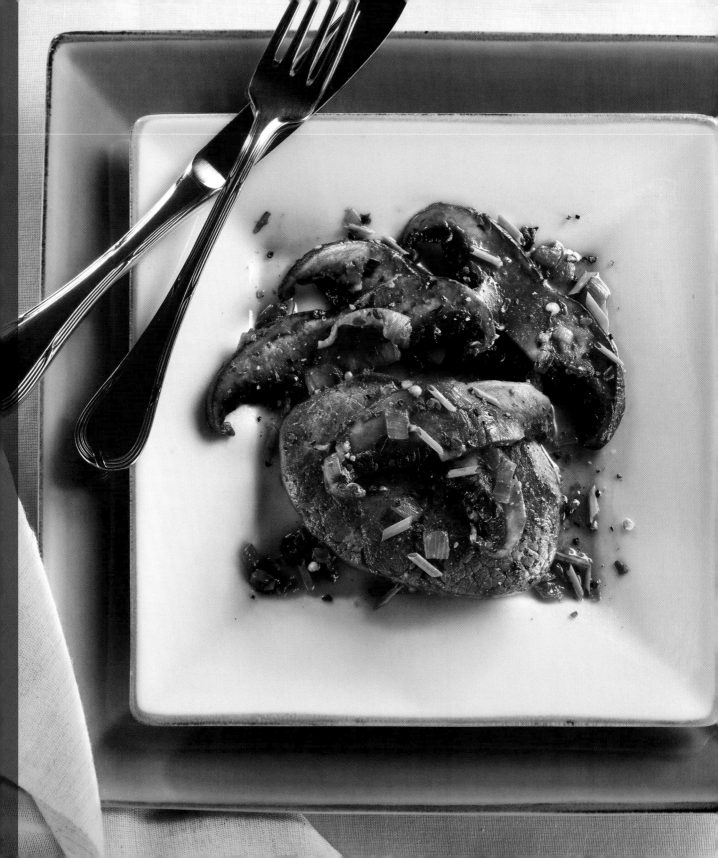

BEEF TENDERLOIN AND PORTOBELLOS
with Marsala Sauce

YIELD 4 servings | **SERVING SIZE** 1 steak + ⅓ cup mushrooms

Marsala wine and spicy pepper flakes elevate this dish to steakhouse quality.

1 package (6 ounces) sliced portobello mushrooms

¼ cup Marsala wine

3 teaspoons canola oil, divided

⅛ teaspoon dried red pepper flakes

½ teaspoon coarsely ground black pepper

¼ teaspoon salt

4 beef tenderloin steaks (4 ounces each)

Canola oil cooking spray

2 large shallots, peeled and finely chopped (2 ounces total)

1 teaspoon low-sodium beef bouillon granules

¼ cup water

1–2 tablespoons fresh chives, sliced diagonally

1 Preheat oven to 200°F.

2 Place mushrooms in a large, resealable plastic bag. Add wine, 2 teaspoons canola oil, and pepper flakes. Seal bag and toss back and forth to coat evenly. Marinate for 15 minutes, turning frequently.

3 Meanwhile, sprinkle black pepper and salt evenly over beef, and let stand 15 minutes at room temperature. Heat 1 teaspoon canola oil in a large nonstick skillet over medium-high heat, tilting to coat bottom lightly. Add beef, cook 4 minutes on one side, turn, and cook 2 minutes or to desired doneness. Put on an oven-proof plate and place in the oven to keep warm.

4 Remove mushrooms from marinade, reserving marinade. Coat pan residue in skillet with cooking spray and cook shallots 30 seconds, stirring constantly. Add mushrooms, coat with cooking spray, and cook 3 minutes or until tender, stirring frequently using two utensils. Add reserved marinade, bouillon granules, and water. Boil for 1 minute to thicken; remove from heat.

5 Place steaks on individual dinner plates. Add any leftover beef juices to mushroom mixture, stir well, and spoon equal amounts over each steak. Sprinkle evenly with chives.

Calories 210	Cholesterol 60 mg	**EXCHANGES PER SERVING**
Calories from fat 80	Sodium 420 mg	½ carbohydrate
Total fat 9.0 g	Total carbohydrate 6 g	3 lean meat
Saturated fat 2.5 g	Dietary fiber 1 g	1 fat
Trans fat 0.0 g	Sugars 2 g	
	Protein 23 g	

RED WINE-BRAISED BEEF WITH VEGETABLES

YIELD 5 servings | **SERVING SIZE** 1 cup

Slow cooking is the lazy way to braise! Simply brown the beef, toss it in a slow cooker with the rest of the ingredients, and have a yummy dinner waiting for you at the end of the day.

Canola oil cooking spray

4 medium parsnips (about 12 ounces total), peeled and cut into 1/2-inch slices, cut large slices in half

3 teaspoons canola oil, divided

1 lb trimmed boneless beef chuck shoulder roast, cut into bite-size pieces

1 large onion (6 ounces), cut into 1/2-inch wedges

4 medium carrots (about 12 ounces), peeled and cut into 1/2-inch slices

1 medium celery stalk, halved lengthwise and cut into 1-inch pieces

2 medium cloves garlic, minced

1 1/2 cups water, divided

1/4 cup dry red wine

1 tablespoon beef bouillon granules

1 teaspoon dried thyme leaves

1/2 teaspoon salt

1 Spray a 3 1/2- or 4-quart slow cooker with cooking spray.

2 Place parsnips in the slow cooker. Heat 1 teaspoon canola oil in a large nonstick skillet over medium-high heat, tilting skillet to coat bottom lightly. Add half of beef and cook 4 minutes or until browned, stirring occasionally. Place in the slow cooker over parsnips. Repeat with 1 teaspoon canola oil and remaining beef.

3 To pan residue in skillet, add remaining 1 teaspoon canola oil, tilting to coat bottom. Add onion, carrots, and celery. Cook 3 minutes or until beginning to brown, stirring occasionally. Add garlic and cook 15 seconds. Remove from heat and pour over beef in slow cooker.

4 To skillet, add 1/2 cup water, wine, bouillon, and thyme. Bring just to a boil over medium-high heat, stirring constantly to blend well. Pour mixture over ingredients in the slow cooker. Cover tightly and cook on high setting 4–4 1/2 hours or on low setting 8–9 hours or until beef is very tender. Add salt and remaining 1 cup water. Stir gently.

Calories 210
  Calories from fat 65
Total fat 7.0 g
  Saturated fat 1.3 g
  Trans fat 0.0 g

Cholesterol 45 mg
Sodium 860 mg
Total carbohydrate 22 g
  Dietary fiber 5 g
  Sugars 7 g
  Protein 16 g

EXCHANGES PER SERVING
1/2 starch
2 vegetable
2 lean meat
1/2 fat

Flavorful tip Be sure to trim all visible fat from the beef and to heat the skillet to ensure proper browning. The skillet is hot if beef sizzles in it. This dish may be served over 3 cups cooked no-yolk egg noodles, if desired.

DRUNKEN BEEF GOULASH

YIELD 4 servings | **SERVING SIZE** 1 cup

Adding a can of beer instead of water or other liquids to this hearty dish gives it personality and a subtle pub-like taste and aroma.

Canola oil cooking spray
1 tablespoon canola oil
³/₄ lb trimmed beef stew meat, cut into 1-inch pieces
1 cup chopped onions
1 cup chopped green pepper
1 package (8 ounces) sliced mushrooms
1 can (12 ounces) lager beer
2 teaspoons Worcestershire sauce
½ teaspoon dried oregano leaves
½ of 6-ounce can tomato paste
1–1¼ teaspoon sugar
½ teaspoon salt

1 Spray a 3½- or 4-quart slow cooker with cooking spray.

2 Heat canola oil in a large nonstick skillet over medium-high heat. Add beef and cook until browned on the edges, about 4 minutes, stirring frequently. Place in the slow cooker and top with onions, pepper, and mushrooms.

3 Add half of beer, Worcestershire sauce, oregano, and tomato paste. Cook and stir for 30 seconds until well blended. Add to slow cooker with remaining beer. Cover tightly and cook on high setting 4½–5 hours or on low setting 9–10 hours until beef is very tender. Add sugar and salt and let stand for 15 minutes for flavors to blend.

Flavorful tip Trim the fat off the beef chuck. Using canola oil instead of the beef fat reduces saturated fat and gives the beef a rich brown color. If desired, serve this dish over 2 cups prepared frozen mashed potatoes, omitting any salt or fat.

Calories 195
Calories from fat 65
Total fat 7.0 g
Saturated fat 1.3 g
Trans fat 0.0 g

Cholesterol 40 mg
Sodium 370 mg
Total carbohydrate 17 g
Dietary fiber 3 g
Sugars 9 g
Protein 17 g

EXCHANGES PER SERVING
½ carbohydrate
2 vegetable
2 lean meat
½ fat

CREAMY BEEF, MUSHROOMS, AND NOODLES

YIELD 4 servings | **SERVING SIZE** ¾ cup beef mixture + ½ cup noodles

This is a healthier version of beef stroganoff. Canola mayonnaise adds moisture, creaminess, and flavor to the dish without guilt.

1 cup (4 ounces) dry no-yolk egg noodles

¼ cup canola mayonnaise

¼ cup dry sherry (or ¼ cup water and 1–2 teaspoons balsamic vinegar)

2 teaspoons beef bouillon granules

1 teaspoon Worcestershire sauce

½ teaspoon coarsely ground black pepper, or to taste

3 teaspoons canola oil, divided

¾ lb boneless sirloin steak, very thinly sliced

1 cup thinly sliced onions

1 package (8 ounces) sliced mushrooms

1 Cook pasta according to package directions, omitting any salt or fat.

2 Meanwhile, whisk together canola mayonnaise, sherry, bouillon, Worcestershire sauce, and black pepper in a medium bowl. Set aside.

3 Heat 1 teaspoon canola oil in a large nonstick skillet over medium-high heat. Tilt skillet to coat bottom lightly. Cook beef 3 minutes and set aside on a separate plate. Heat 1 teaspoon canola oil, add onions, and cook 5 minutes or until just beginning to richly brown, stirring frequently. Scrape onions to one side of the skillet, add remaining 1 teaspoon canola oil, and add mushrooms. Cook 4 minutes or until mushrooms begin to brown on the edges, stirring frequently. Add beef and any accumulated juices. Cook 30 seconds or until most of the liquid has evaporated.

4 Remove from heat and stir in canola mayonnaise mixture until well blended. Serve over drained noodles. Sprinkle with additional black pepper, if desired.

Calories 320	Cholesterol 30 mg	**EXCHANGES PER SERVING**
Calories from fat 110	Sodium 615 mg	1½ starch
Total fat 12.0 g	Total carbohydrate 27 g	1 vegetable
Saturated fat 1.5 g	Dietary fiber 2 g	3 lean meat
Trans fat 0.1 g	Sugars 4 g	1 fat
	Protein 23 g	

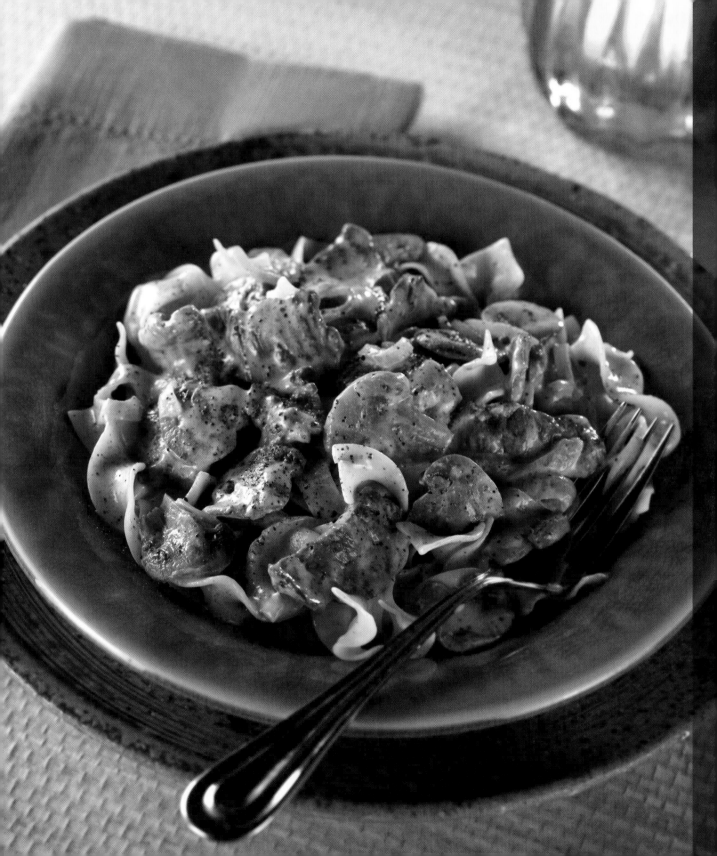

LAYERED MEXICAN CASSEROLE

YIELD 4 servings | **SERVING SIZE** 1 cup

Mexican-style cuisine is always popular. Combining small amounts of beef with beans, brown rice, and reduced-fat cheese in this dish controls unwanted fat calories while providing protein and great taste.

¾ cup quick-cooking brown rice

3 teaspoons canola oil, divided

½ lb 96% lean ground beef

½ cup finely chopped onion

½ of 1-ounce package (or 1 tablespoon) taco seasoning mix

½ of 16-ounce can dark kidney beans, rinsed and drained

½ cup water

2 tablespoons canola mayonnaise

⅓ cup fat-free sour cream

¼ cup chopped fresh cilantro leaves

1 ounce reduced-fat sharp cheddar cheese, grated or shredded

Fresh tomatoes, for garnish

1 medium lime, quartered

1 Preheat oven to 350°F. Cook rice according to package directions.

2 Meanwhile, heat 1 teaspoon canola oil in a large nonstick skillet over medium-high heat. Tilt skillet to coat bottom lightly. Cook beef for 2 minutes, stirring constantly. Add remaining 2 teaspoons canola oil and onion to beef. Cook for 3 minutes or until onion is translucent, stirring frequently. Remove from heat, add taco seasoning, and stir until well blended. Stir in beans and ½ cup water until mixed well. Cover to keep warm.

3 Remove rice from heat. Toss rice with canola mayonnaise and then with sour cream. Spoon into the bottom of a 9-inch, deep-dish pie pan, and sprinkle evenly with cilantro. Spoon beef mixture on top and sprinkle evenly with cheese. Bake, uncovered, for 15 minutes to heat through. Top with fresh tomatoes and serve with lime wedges.

Calories 355
 Calories from fat 100
Total fat 11.0 g
 Saturated fat 2.2 g
 Trans fat 0.2 g

Cholesterol 35 mg
Sodium 500 mg
Total carbohydrate 42 g
 Dietary fiber 4 g
 Sugars 4 g
Protein 22 g

EXCHANGES PER SERVING

3 starch

2 lean meat

1 fat

BARLEY, WHITE BEAN, AND ARTICHOKE TOSS

YIELD 4 servings | **SERVING SIZE** 1 cup

In a matter of minutes, you can sit down and enjoy basil-infused barley and white beans tossed with toasted pine nuts, skillet-roasted artichokes, and creamy feta cheese!

1⅓ cups water

⅔ cup quick-cooking barley

½ of 15-ounce can navy beans, rinsed and drained

3 teaspoons canola oil, divided

¼ cup (1 ounce) pine nuts

½ of 14-ounce can quartered artichokes, drained and patted dry

2 tablespoons chopped fresh basil leaves

⅓ cup (1½ ounces) crumbled reduced-fat feta cheese, divided

1 medium clove garlic, minced

¼ teaspoon salt

1 medium tomato, seeded and diced, or 1 cup grape tomatoes, quartered

1 Bring water to a boil in a medium saucepan. Add barley and return to a boil. Reduce heat and simmer, covered, 10 minutes or until tender. Add beans to barley during last 2 minutes of cooking, then drain.

2 Meanwhile, heat a large nonstick skillet over medium-high heat. Add pine nuts and cook for 1–2 minutes or until lightly toasted, stirring constantly. Set aside on a separate plate. Heat 1 teaspoon canola oil in the skillet. Tilt skillet to coat bottom lightly, add artichokes, and cook 3 minutes to brown. Remove from heat and add barley mixture, 2 teaspoons canola oil, basil, half of feta, toasted pine nuts, garlic, and salt. Top with tomatoes and remaining feta.

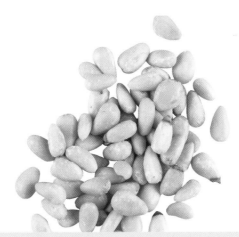

Fresh tip Be sure to pat the artichokes dry with paper towels; otherwise, they will stew instead of brown.

Calories 255
  Calories from fat 90
Total fat 10.0 g
  Saturated fat 1.6 g
  Trans fat 0.0 g

Cholesterol 5 mg
Sodium 445 mg
Total carbohydrate 34 g
  Dietary fiber 6 g
  Sugars 3 g
Protein 9 g

EXCHANGES PER SERVING
1½ starch
1 vegetable
2 fat

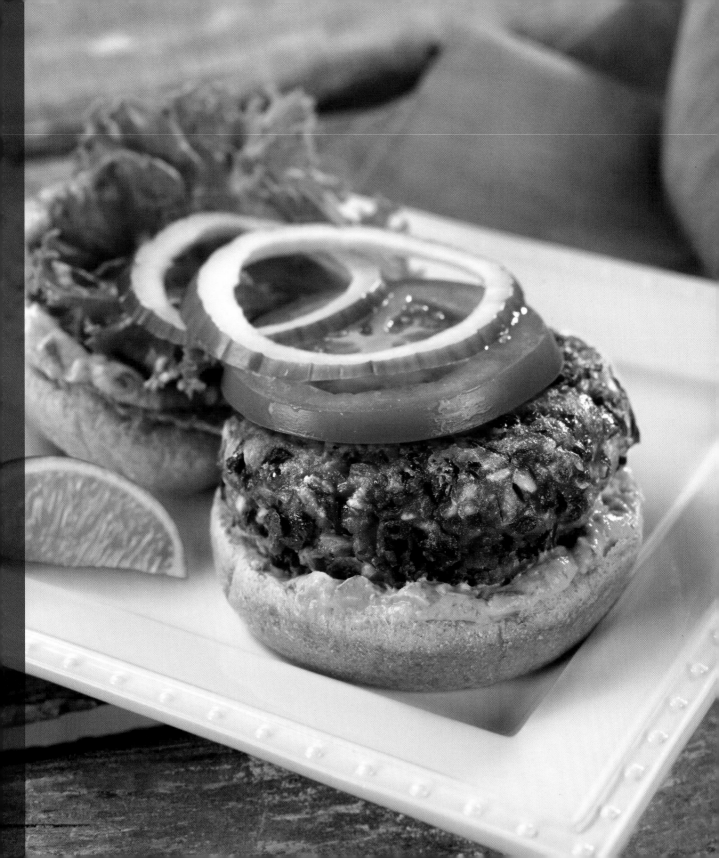

BLACK BEAN BURGERS
with Avocado-Lime Mayonnaise

YIELD 4 servings | **SERVING SIZE** 1 burger

Jazz up these yummy burgers with avocado-lime canola mayonnaise and you'll have a vegetarian dish that even the biggest meat eaters you know can't resist.

MAYONNAISE

- ½ ripe medium avocado, peeled and pitted
- 2 tablespoons canola mayonnaise
- 1 tablespoon fresh lime juice
- 1 tablespoon water
- ¼ cup chopped fresh cilantro leaves

BURGERS

- 1 can (15 ounces) black beans, rinsed and drained
- ½ of 15-ounce can dark kidney beans, rinsed and drained
- ½ cup finely chopped green bell pepper
- ⅓ cup quick-cooking oats
- 2 large egg whites
- 1 tablespoon canola oil
- ⅛–¼ teaspoon cayenne pepper

  Canola oil cooking spray
- 4 whole-wheat hamburger buns, split and toasted
- ¼ cup thinly sliced red onion
- 4 tomato slices
- 4 lettuce leaves
- 4 lime wedges (optional)

1 Place canola mayonnaise ingredients in a blender, secure lid, and purée until smooth.

2 Place beans in a gallon-size resealable bag. Using a meat mallet, pound beans to a coarse texture, until they resemble lumpy mashed potatoes. Place beans in a medium bowl and add bell pepper, oats, egg whites, canola oil, and cayenne pepper. Mix well and shape into four patties.

3 Coat a large nonstick skillet with cooking spray and heat over medium heat. Add patties and cook 4 minutes on each side or until they begin to lightly brown. The patties will be fragile, so be sure to turn them gently.

4 To assemble, spoon 1 tablespoon canola mayonnaise mixture on each bun half. Top each bottom bun with burger, onion, a tomato slice, and a lettuce leaf. Place bun tops over each. Serve with lime wedges.

Fresh tip If desired, omit the buns and serve the patties on the lettuce leaf, tomato slice, and onion. Spoon the mayonnaise mixture on top of the patties and serve with lime wedges.

Calories 300
  Calories from fat 110
Total fat 12.0 g
  Saturated fat 1.8 g
  Trans fat 0.0 g

Cholesterol 0 mg
Sodium 785 mg
Total carbohydrate 33 g
  Dietary fiber 10 g
  Sugars 5 g
Protein 19 g

EXCHANGES PER SERVING
2 starch
2 lean meat
1 fat

BLACK BEAN SKILLET
with Butternut Squash

YIELD 4 servings | **SERVING SIZE** 1 squash quarter + 1 cup bean mixture

With this speedy skillet recipe, you can cook the squash in about 10 minutes and finish it off with a nutritious, flavorful topping instead of butter.

3 teaspoons canola oil, divided

1 cup chopped onions

1 medium Anaheim chile pepper, sliced in rounds (seeded, if desired)

1¼ cups water, divided

¾ cup quick-cooking brown rice

1 can (15 ounces) black beans, rinsed and drained

1 can (10 ounces) mild tomatoes with chiles

⅛ teaspoon ground turmeric (optional)

1 medium butternut squash (about 1½ lbs), quartered, seeded, and skin pierced several times with a fork

½ cup fat-free sour cream

2–3 tablespoons chopped fresh cilantro leaves

1 Heat 2 teaspoons canola oil in a large nonstick skillet over medium-high heat. Tilt skillet to coat bottom lightly. Cook onions 4 minutes or until they begin to brown on the edges, stirring frequently. Scrape onions to one side of skillet, add 1 teaspoon canola oil, then add peppers and cook 2 minutes. Add 1 cup water, rice, beans, tomatoes, and turmeric. Bring to a boil over medium-high heat, reduce heat, cover tightly, and simmer 12 minutes or until rice is tender.

2 Meanwhile, place squash and remaining ¼ cup water in a microwave-safe shallow pan (such as a 9-inch, deep-dish pie pan), cover, and microwave on high 10 minutes or until tender when pierced with a fork. Drain.

3 To serve, place squash quarter on each of four dinner plates, and spoon equal amounts of bean mixture on each squash wedge. Top with sour cream and cilantro.

Calories 345
   Calories from fat 45
Total fat 5.0 g
   Saturated fat 0.4 g
   Trans fat 0.0 g

Cholesterol 5 mg
Sodium 410 mg
Total carbohydrate 63 g
   Dietary fiber 9 g
   Sugars 9 g
   Protein 13 g

EXCHANGES PER SERVING
3½ starch
1 vegetable
½ fat

Flavorful tip Adding the canola oil in stages helps to brown the various ingredients without adding too much fat. This dish may be served without the squash, if desired.

SWEET HOME CHILI ON SPAGHETTI SQUASH

YIELD 4 servings | **SERVING SIZE** 1 cup chili + ½ cup squash

Adding a small amount of sugar to this dish softens the acidic taste of the tomatoes without too much sweetness. Spaghetti squash is always fun to make and here it replaces pasta.

1 medium spaghetti squash (about 2½ lbs)

1 tablespoon canola oil

1 cup diced onions

1 cup diced green pepper

1 can (14.5 ounces) stewed tomatoes

1 can (15.5 ounces) pinto beans, rinsed and drained

1 cup brewed coffee (or 1 cup water + 1 teaspoon instant coffee granules)

2 teaspoons chili powder

1 teaspoon ground cumin, divided

1½ teaspoons sugar

½ cup fat-free sour cream

½ cup (2 ounces) shredded reduced-fat sharp cheddar cheese

2–3 tablespoons chopped fresh cilantro leaves

1 Poke several holes in the skin of the squash with a fork and microwave on high for 10 minutes. Squash should be tender when pierced with a fork; if it isn't, microwave on high in 1-minute intervals until tender. Let sit to cool slightly. When squash is cool enough to handle, cut in half and discard seeds. Scrape inside with the fork to remove spaghetti-like strands. Transfer to a heat-proof serving dish and keep warm.

2 Meanwhile, heat canola oil in a Dutch oven over medium-high heat. Add onions and pepper and cook for 5 minutes or until they begin to richly brown. Add tomatoes, beans, coffee, chili powder, and ½ teaspoon cumin. Bring to a boil over high heat. Reduce heat and simmer, covered, for 20 minutes or until tomatoes are tender and mixture has thickened. Break up any large pieces of tomato with the back of a spoon near the end of the cooking time. Remove from heat and add remaining ½ teaspoon cumin and sugar.

3 To serve, place in bowls and top with chili, then sour cream, cheese, and cilantro.

Fast tip Roasted squash seeds are a healthy snack. To make them, wash the seeds and place them in an oven-proof dish sprayed with canola oil cooking spray. Season as you prefer, then roast for 7–10 minutes at 400°F, cool, and serve.

Calories 295	Cholesterol 15 mg
Calories from fat 70	Sodium 525 mg
Total fat 8.0 g	Total carbohydrate 43 g
Saturated fat 2.3 g	Dietary fiber 11 g
Trans fat 0.0 g	Sugars 14 g
	Protein 15 g

EXCHANGES PER SERVING

2 starch
2 vegetable
1 lean meat
1 fat

VEGETABLE PASTA
with Tapenade and Pine Nuts

YIELD 4 servings | **SERVING SIZE** 1 cup pasta and beans + ¹⁄₂ cup vegetables

This dish is layered with flavor and texture from the smoky roasted vegetables, the intense flavors of the olives and fresh basil, the tender white beans, and pasta!

VEGETABLE PASTA

Canola oil cooking spray

1 medium zucchini, quartered lengthwise and cut into 2-inch pieces

1 medium green bell pepper, cut into 1-inch pieces

1 cup grape tomatoes

1 teaspoon canola oil

¹⁄₄ cup (1 ounce) pine nuts

¹⁄₄ teaspoon salt

2 cups (6 ounces) dry whole-grain penne pasta

¹⁄₂ of 15-ounce can navy beans, rinsed and drained, or ¹⁄₈ of 16-ounce package cubed silken super-firm tofu

TAPENADE

¹⁄₄ cup chopped fresh basil leaves (or ¹⁄₄ cup chopped fresh parsley and 1 tablespoon plus 1 teaspoon dried basil leaves)

12 pitted kalamata olives, finely chopped

2 medium cloves garlic, minced

2 tablespoons water

2–3 teaspoons red wine vinegar

1 tablespoon canola oil

¹⁄₄ teaspoon salt

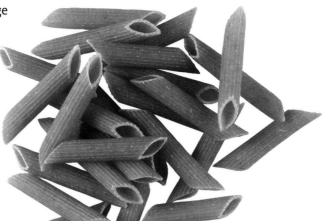

Fast tip To boil pasta water faster, use hot tap water and cover it with a lid.

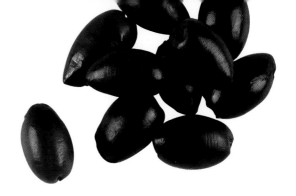

1 Preheat oven to 425°F. Line a large baking sheet with foil and coat with cooking spray.

2 Place zucchini, bell pepper, and tomatoes on the prepared baking sheet; drizzle with 1 teaspoon canola oil. Toss to coat lightly and arrange in a single layer. Bake 15 minutes, sprinkle pine nuts on the baking sheet between vegetables, and bake 4 more minutes or until vegetables are richly browned on the edges. Watch carefully so the nuts do not burn. Remove from oven, sprinkle with ¼ teaspoon salt, wrap foil up around vegetables, sealing tightly, and let stand 10 minutes to absorb flavors.

3 Meanwhile, cook pasta according to package directions, omitting any salt or fat, and add beans or tofu during last minute of cooking.

4 Combine tapenade ingredients in a small bowl. Drain pasta mixture and shake off excess liquid. Place on a serving platter or shallow pasta bowl, spoon tapenade over pasta, and top with vegetables. Sprinkle with additional basil, if desired.

Calories 325
   Calories from fat 110
Total fat 12.0 g
   Saturated fat 1.0 g
   Trans fat 0.0 g

Cholesterol 0 mg
Sodium 470 mg
Total carbohydrate 48 g
   Dietary fiber 9 g
   Sugars 5 g
Protein 10 g

EXCHANGES PER SERVING
2½ starch
1 vegetable
2 fat

CURRIED SWEET POTATO AND PEANUT STEW

YIELD 4 servings | **SERVING SIZE** 1⅓ cups

This stew is perfect year-round, although it's most appreciated on a cold winter night!

- 1 tablespoon canola oil
- 1 cup diced onions
- 3 medium sweet potatoes (1 lb), peeled and cut into ½-inch cubes
- ½ of 15.5-ounce can chickpeas, rinsed and drained
- ½ of 16-ounce can dark kidney beans, rinsed and drained
- 1 can (14.5 ounces) diced tomatoes
- 1 can (14 ounces) vegetable broth
- 3 tablespoons reduced-fat peanut butter
- 1½ teaspoons sugar
- 1½ teaspoons ground cumin
- ½ teaspoon curry powder or ground cinnamon
- ¼ teaspoon black pepper
- ⅛ teaspoon cayenne pepper
- ¼ cup chopped fresh cilantro leaves

1 Heat canola oil in a Dutch oven over medium-high heat. Add onions and cook 6 minutes or until they are richly browned, stirring frequently.

2 Add potatoes and cook 2 minutes. Add remaining ingredients, except cilantro, and bring to a boil over high heat. Reduce heat, cover, and simmer 25–30 minutes or until potatoes are very tender. Spoon into bowls and serve topped with cilantro.

Calories 335	Cholesterol 0 mg
Calories from fat 80	Sodium 805 mg
Total fat 9.0 g	Total carbohydrate 52 g
Saturated fat 1.2 g	Dietary fiber 10 g
Trans fat 0.0 g	Sugars 18 g
	Protein 12 g

EXCHANGES PER SERVING
2½ starch
2 vegetable
1½ fat

Flavorful tip Be sure to cook the onions the full 6 minutes to ensure rich, brown results.

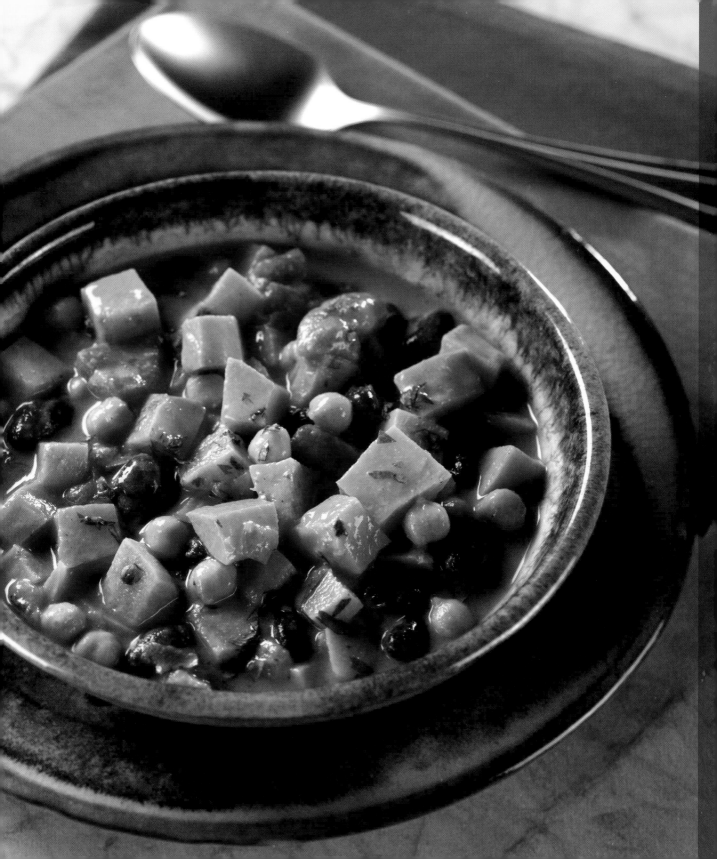

TOASTED PECAN QUINOA WITH RED PEPPERS

YIELD 4 servings | **SERVING SIZE** 1 cup

Quinoa was a staple of the ancient Incans and it contains more protein than any other grain. Combined with vegetables, nuts, and raisins, this dish explodes with texture and nutrients.

1½ cups water

¾ cup quick-cooking quinoa

½ teaspoon curry powder

⅛ teaspoon cayenne pepper (optional)

½ cup golden raisins

½ cup (2 ounces) chopped pecans

3 teaspoons canola oil, divided

1 cup diced onions

1 cup diced red bell pepper

½ teaspoon salt

1 Bring water to a boil in a medium saucepan over high heat. Add quinoa, curry powder, and cayenne pepper; then reduce heat, cover, and cook 7 minutes. Add raisins and continue to cook, covered, 3–4 minutes or until liquid is absorbed.

2 Meanwhile, heat a large nonstick skillet over medium-high heat. Add pecans and cook 1–2 minutes or until they begin to brown, stirring constantly. Remove from the skillet and set aside on a separate plate.

3 In the same skillet, heat 1 teaspoon canola oil over medium-high heat. Tilt skillet to coat bottom lightly. Add onions and cook 4 minutes or until they begin to richly brown, stirring frequently. Add bell pepper and cook 2 minutes, stirring frequently.

4 Remove from heat. Add quinoa, salt, and half of pecans. Toss to blend. Sprinkle evenly with remaining pecans and drizzle remaining 2 teaspoons canola oil over all. Do not stir. Let stand 5 minutes before serving.

		EXCHANGES PER SERVING	
Calories 340	Cholesterol 0 mg		*Flavorful tip* It's important not to stir in the canola oil, so it can better pull out the richness of the other flavors, especially from the nuts. For extra protein, add ½ cup diced tofu or black beans to the dish.
Calories from fat 145	Sodium 305 mg	1½ starch	
Total fat 16.0 g	Total carbohydrate 45 g	1 fruit	
Saturated fat 1.5 g	Dietary fiber 6 g	1 vegetable	
Trans fat 0.0 g	Sugars 18 g	3 fat	
	Protein 7 g		

SESAME THAI TOSS WITH PEANUT LIME SAUCE

YIELD 4 servings | **SERVING SIZE** 1½ cups

Health professionals recommend getting healthy unsaturated fat from such sources as nuts, seeds, and canola oil, and this dish has them all! Savor the distinctive flavor of the peanut butter in the sauce.

SAUCE

- 3 tablespoons reduced-fat peanut butter
- 3 tablespoons reduced-sodium soy sauce
- 3 tablespoons fresh lime juice
- 3 tablespoons water
- 1½ tablespoons pourable sugar substitute
- ¼ teaspoon dried red pepper flakes (optional)
- 2 teaspoons canola oil

NOODLES

- ½ of 13.25-ounce package whole-grain spaghetti or dry soba noodles
- ¾ cup frozen green peas
- 1 tablespoon sesame seeds
- 1 teaspoon canola oil
- 1 cup matchstick carrots
- ½ medium red bell pepper, thinly sliced and cut into 2-inch pieces
- ¾ cup finely chopped whole green onions
- ½ cup chopped fresh cilantro leaves

1 Place peanut butter and soy sauce in a small microwave-safe bowl and microwave for 20–25 seconds on high. Whisk until well blended and stir in remaining sauce ingredients. Set aside.

2 Cook pasta according to package directions, omitting any salt and fat. Add frozen peas during last 30 seconds of cooking.

3 Heat a large nonstick skillet over medium-high heat. Add sesame seeds and cook 1–2 minutes or until lightly toasted, stirring frequently. Set aside on a separate plate. Add 1 teaspoon canola oil to skillet and tilt to coat bottom lightly. Add carrots and bell pepper and cook 2 minutes or until slightly limp, stirring frequently. Remove from heat.

4 Place drained noodle mixture in a shallow bowl. Spoon sauce evenly over noodles, sprinkle with sesame seeds, and top with vegetables from skillet. Sprinkle onions and cilantro on top. Serve as is or gently tossed.

Calories 280
    Calories from fat 80
Total fat 9.0 g
    Saturated fat 1.2 g
    Trans fat 0.0 g

Cholesterol 0 mg
Sodium 600 mg
Total carbohydrate 41 g
    Dietary fiber 5 g
    Sugars 8 g
Protein 12 g

EXCHANGES PER SERVING
2 starch
1 vegetable
2 fat

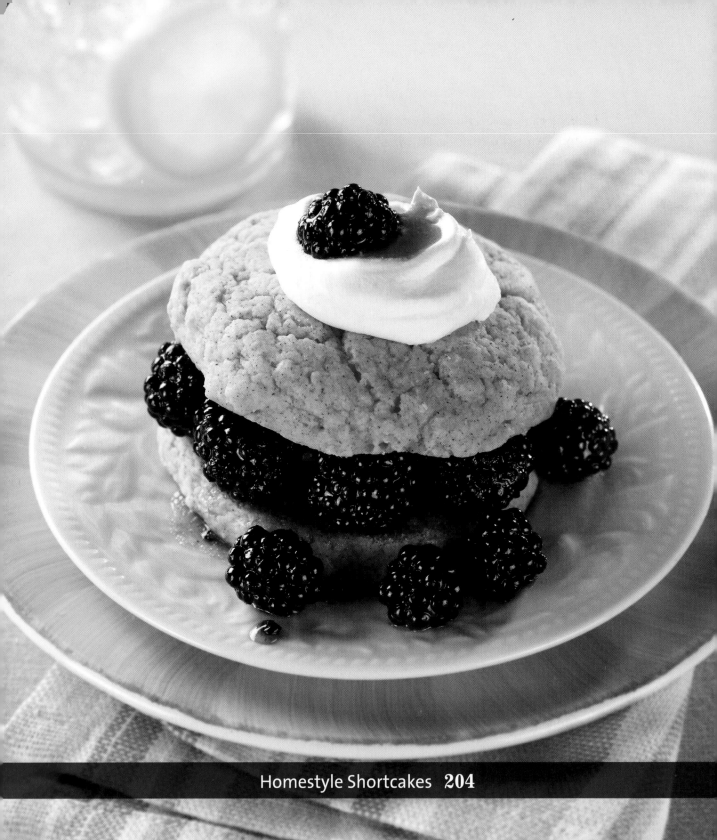

DESSERTS

Glazed Pineapple-Orange Bundt Cake | **194**

Mini Fruit Tarts with Cheesecake Filling | **195**

Mango-Banana Phyllo Nests | **196**

Harvest Pumpkin Pie | **198**

Chocolate Mint Pie with Espresso Sauce | **199**

Skillet Pie with Oat-Pecan Crumble | **200**

Fresh and Dried Fruit Ginger Crumble | **201**

Blueberry-Lemon Country Cobbler | **203**

Homestyle Shortcakes | **204**

Spiced Berry Sauce | **205**

Melon Infused with Mint and Lime | **206**

Traditional Rolled Sugar Cookies | **207**

Toffee-Pecan Topped Cookies | **208**

Sticky, Crunchy Cereal Rounds | **210**

Apricot-Cranberry Nut Squares | **211**

Rich, Warm Brownie Wedges
with Java Cream | **212**

Chocolate Fondue | **214**

GLAZED PINEAPPLE-ORANGE BUNDT CAKE

YIELD 16 servings | **SERVING SIZE** 1 slice

This dense cake bursts with tropical flavors. It's no ordinary Bundt cake!

CAKE
Canola oil cooking spray

1¼ cups all-purpose flour, spooned into measuring cups and leveled

1 cup plus 2 tablespoons white whole-wheat flour, spooned into measuring cup and leveled

2½ teaspoons baking powder

½ teaspoon salt

½ teaspoon ground nutmeg

¾ cup packed brown sugar substitute blend

⅓ cup canola oil

2 teaspoons vanilla extract

½ cup egg substitute

1⅓ cups water

1 tablespoon orange zest

1 can (20 ounces) crushed pineapple in its own juice, drained

GLAZE
½ cup orange juice

2 teaspoons cornstarch

½ cup sweetened coconut (optional)

1 Preheat oven to 325°F. Coat a nonstick Bundt pan with cooking spray and set aside. Combine flours, baking powder, salt, and nutmeg in a medium bowl and set aside.

2 Add sugar, canola oil, and vanilla in a large bowl. Using an electric mixer on medium-high speed, beat until well blended. Add egg substitute, water, and zest, and beat until well blended. Reduce mixer to low speed and gradually add flour mixture until just combined.

3 Spoon drained pineapple into the bottom of the Bundt pan and pour batter evenly over all. Bake 55 minutes or until a wooden pick inserted in center comes out clean. Transfer cake (still in pan) to a cooling rack. Let cool 20 minutes, then invert onto a serving plate. Let cool completely, at least 1 hour.

4 Meanwhile, combine orange juice and cornstarch in a small saucepan. Stir until completely dissolved. Bring to a boil over medium-high heat and continue boiling for 1 minute. Remove from heat and let cool completely.

5 When cake and glaze have cooled, spoon sauce evenly over top of cake, using the back of a spoon to spread down sides slightly. Sprinkle evenly with coconut. Store leftovers covered in plastic wrap in the refrigerator or freeze in individual slices for portion control.

Calories 180
  Calories from fat 45
Total fat 5.0 g
  Saturated fat 1.0 g
  Trans fat 0.0 g

Cholesterol 0 mg
Sodium 155 mg
Total carbohydrate 29 g
  Dietary fiber 2 g
  Sugars 14 g
Protein 3 g

EXCHANGES PER SERVING
2 carbohydrate
1 fat

MINI FRUIT TARTS
with Cheesecake Filling

YIELD 6 servings | **SERVING SIZE** 1 tart

These individual cheesecake cups are easy to make, easy to store, and very easy to enjoy.

Canola oil cooking spray

CRUST

- ³/₄ cup graham cracker crumbs
- 1¹/₂ tablespoons canola oil
- 2 tablespoons honey

FILLING

- 2 ounces light whipped cream cheese, soft tub variety, softened
- ²/₃ cup fat-free sour cream
- 1 teaspoon vanilla extract
- 1¹/₂ tablespoons pourable sugar substitute
- 1¹/₂ teaspoons fresh lemon juice
- ¹/₄ teaspoon lemon zest

TOPPING

- 2 ripe medium kiwi, peeled and diced
- 1 can (8 ounces) pineapple tidbits, packed in juice, well drained

1 Preheat oven to 350°F.

2 Coat six 6-ounce glass or ceramic ramekins with cooking spray. Combine crumbs, canola oil, and honey in a medium bowl and stir until mixture achieves a crumb consistency. Spoon equal amounts (about 3 tablespoons) into each ramekin. Press down with the back of a spoon or your thumbs to form a crust on the bottom and up the sides slightly. Place on a baking sheet and bake 6 minutes or until slightly golden and fragrant. Place the baking sheet on a wire rack to cool completely. (Crust will not be set at this point. It will harden as it cools.)

3 When crusts have cooled, combine filling ingredients in another medium bowl. To soften cream cheese, place it in a bowl and microwave on high for 15 seconds. Using an electric mixer on the medium-high setting, beat mixture until smooth. Spoon equal amounts (about 2 tablespoons) of cream cheese mixture into each ramekin. Top with equal amounts of kiwi and pineapple.

Fast tip When measuring honey or maple syrup, coat a spoon with canola oil spray or, if canola oil is in the recipe, measure the oil before the honey. The honey will slide off the oil and not stick.

Calories 175
Calories from fat 65
Total fat 7.0 g
    Saturated fat 1.5 g
    Trans fat 0.0 g

Cholesterol 10 mg
Sodium 120 mg
Total carbohydrate 24 g
    Dietary fiber 2 g
    Sugars 17 g
Protein 4 g

EXCHANGES PER SERVING
1¹/₂ carbohydrate
1¹/₂ fat

MANGO-BANANA PHYLLO NESTS

YIELD 6 servings | **SERVING SIZE** 1 phyllo nest

This show-stopping dessert will win you compliments every single time you serve it. It will look as though you went to a lot of effort...effortlessly!

CRUST

1 tablespoon canola oil

6 sheets frozen phyllo dough, thawed

FILLING

1½ teaspoons canola oil

2 tablespoons packed brown sugar substitute blend

1 tablespoon orange juice

1 ripe mango, peeled, seeded, and diced

1 medium banana, peeled, quartered lengthwise, and diced

2 tablespoons confectioner's sugar

¼ cup dark rum (optional)

1 Preheat oven to 350°F. Using 1 tablespoon canola oil, lightly brush one side of each phyllo sheet. Cut each sheet with a sharp knife into four lengthwise strips and then cut each strip in half to make eight squares per sheet.

2 In six alternating cups of a 12-cup muffin pan, lace eight squares of phyllo per cup, oil side up, corners overlapping in the center. (There is not enough room to fill all 12 cups; six is manageable.) Press down gently to allow bottoms to take the shape of the muffin cup. Ruffle edges to create a nest appearance. Repeat with remaining five whole phyllo sheets. Place on a center oven rack and bake 5 minutes or until golden. Remove from oven and place muffin tin on a wire rack to cool completely.

3 Meanwhile, combine remaining 1½ teaspoons canola oil, brown sugar, and orange juice in a medium bowl. Add mango and banana and toss gently, yet thoroughly, to coat.

4 To serve, place phyllo nests on individual dessert plates and spoon equal amounts of mango mixture, about ⅓ cup, into each nest. Place confectioner's sugar in a fine-mesh sieve and sprinkle evenly over the edges of each nest. Spoon 2 teaspoons rum over each. Serve immediately.

Calories 175
Calories from fat 40
Total fat 4.5 g
Saturated fat 0.3 g
Trans fat 0.0 g

Cholesterol 0 mg
Sodium 95 mg
Total carbohydrate 33 g
Dietary fiber 2 g
Sugars 15 g
Protein 2 g

EXCHANGES PER SERVING
2 carbohydrate
1 fat

Fast tip The nests may be prepared 24 hours in advance. Store them carefully in gallon-size, resealable plastic bags at room temperature. Do not fill the nests with the fruit mixture until the time of serving.

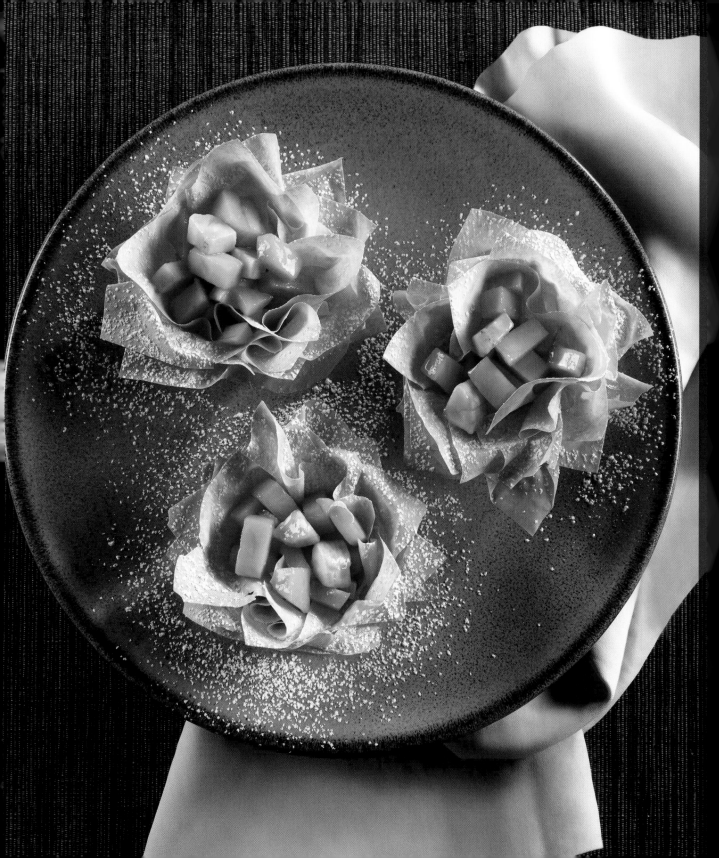

HARVEST PUMPKIN PIE

YIELD 10 servings | **SERVING SIZE** 1 pie slice

For a healthy twist on an old favorite, this recipe uses white whole-wheat flour, canola oil, and almonds in the crust. Harvest fiber and healthy fat.

CRUST

- ¼ cup (1 ounce) slivered almonds
- 1¼ cups white whole-wheat flour, spooned into measuring cups and leveled
- ¼ teaspoon salt
- ¼ teaspoon baking powder
- ⅓ cup canola oil, chilled in the freezer for 2 hours
- 1 egg white
- 2 tablespoons ice water
- 2 tablespoons 1% milk
- 1½ teaspoons cider vinegar

FILLING

- 1 can (15 ounces) solid pumpkin
- ⅔ cup sugar
- 1¼ cups fat-free half and half
- ¾ cup egg substitute
- 2 teaspoons vanilla extract
- ¼ teaspoon salt
- 1 tablespoon pumpkin pie spice (or 2 teaspoons ground cinnamon, ½ teaspoon ground nutmeg, and ½ teaspoon ground ginger)

1 Preheat oven to 375°F. Put almonds in a food processor and pulse once or twice until coarsely ground. Add flour, salt, and baking powder to food processor and pulse once or twice to combine ingredients. Add cold canola oil. Pulse once or twice again.

2 Combine egg white, water, milk, and vinegar in a small bowl. With food processor running, pour liquid ingredients through the feed tube. Turn off machine as soon as ingredients are mixed, about 10 seconds. Remove dough and place on a lightly floured surface. Knead ingredients 4 or 5 times to finish mixing. Roll out to fit a 9-inch, deep-dish pie pan. Trim and flute edges.

3 Combine filling ingredients in a medium bowl and stir until well blended. Fill crust with pie filling, cover edges with foil, and bake 25 minutes. Remove foil and bake another 25 minutes or until a knife inserted near the center comes out clean. Cool on a wire rack. Refrigerate within 2 hours.

Calories 240	Cholesterol 0 mg
Calories from fat 90	Sodium 200 mg
Total fat 10.0 g	Total carbohydrate 33 g
Saturated fat 1.1 g	Dietary fiber 4 g
Trans fat 0.0 g	Sugars 17 g
	Protein 6 g

EXCHANGES PER SERVING
2 carbohydrate
2 fat

Fast tip Keep several portions of canola oil in the freezer for whenever you are ready to make pastry.

CHOCOLATE MINT PIE
with Espresso Sauce

YIELD 10 servings | SERVING SIZE 1 pie slice + 1/4 cup fruit

Chocolate lovers, peppermint lovers, and coffee lovers will unite with this decadent dessert made with a minted chocolate crust, chocolate frozen yogurt, and a bold coffee sauce. Even better news is that you can make it ahead of time!

FILLING

4 cups chocolate no-sugar-added frozen yogurt

CRUST

15 thin chocolate wafers

3 large or 9 small (4 1/2 ounces) chocolate-covered peppermint patties, broken into bite-size pieces

1 tablespoon canola oil

TOPPING

1/2 cup water

3/4 teaspoon cornstarch

1 1/2 teaspoons instant coffee granules

2 1/2 cups frozen dark sweet cherries or unsweetened raspberries, partially thawed

1 Place frozen yogurt container on a counter and let stand 15–20 minutes to soften slightly.

2 Meanwhile, place wafers in a food processor with a metal blade. Process wafers until fine crumbs form. With machine running, add patties one at a time, processing until well blended. Continue processing, adding canola oil to create a coarse crumble texture. Lightly press cookie mixture evenly over the bottom of an 8 1/2- or 9-inch springform pan or deep-dish pie pan. Lightly spoon frozen yogurt on top of cookie mixture. Using the back of a spoon or fork, spread gently to smooth. Cover with plastic wrap and place in the freezer overnight or for at least 8 hours, until firm.

3 To make topping, whisk together water and cornstarch in a small saucepan until completely dissolved. Stir in coffee granules, bring to a boil over high heat, and continue boiling for 1 full minute. Remove from heat and cool completely. Store in a small jar with a lid and refrigerate until needed. When serving, cut pie into 10 wedges, place on a dessert plate, spoon 1 tablespoon espresso topping over each wedge and top with berries. You can store this dish in the freezer for up to one week.

Fast tip Adding canola oil to the pie crust prevents it from becoming too hard, so it is easy to cut when you're ready to serve.

Calories 235	Cholesterol 5 mg
Calories from fat 40	Sodium 130 mg
Total fat 4.5 g	Total carbohydrate 45 g
Saturated fat 1.5 g	Dietary fiber 3 g
Trans fat 0.0 g	Sugars 30 g
	Protein 5 g

EXCHANGES PER SERVING
3 carbohydrate
1/2 fat

SKILLET PIE WITH OAT-PECAN CRUMBLE

YIELD 8 servings | **SERVING SIZE** ½ cup pie

There's no need to heat up the oven for this scrumptious apple and peach pie. It's cooked on top of the stove!

CRUMBLE

- 2 ounces chopped pecan pieces
- ½ cup rolled oats
- 2 tablespoons wheat germ
- ½ teaspoon apple pie spice
- ⅛ teaspoon salt
- 2 tablespoons canola oil
- 2 tablespoons packed dark brown sugar

FILLING

- 1½ lbs Gala apples, peeled, halved, cored, and sliced
- 8 ounces fresh peaches, chopped, or frozen unsweetened peach slices, thawed and chopped
- ⅓ cup packed dark brown sugar
- 1 teaspoon apple pie spice
- 1 tablespoon cornstarch
- ¼ cup water
- 1 teaspoon vanilla extract

1 Combine all crumble ingredients, except the canola oil and sugar, in a medium mixing bowl. Stir to blend thoroughly.

2 Heat canola oil in a medium nonstick skillet over medium heat. Tilt skillet to coat bottom evenly. Sprinkle oat mixture evenly over bottom of skillet, stir to blend, and cook 2 minutes, stirring occasionally. Add sugar and cook 1 minute or until slightly fragrant, but no longer than 1 minute, stirring constantly. Remove skillet from heat and place mixture on a separate plate.

3 To skillet, add apples, peaches, sugar, and spice. Combine cornstarch and water in another small bowl, then stir into skillet mixture until cornstarch is completely dissolved. Place over medium-high heat, bring to a boil, and continue to boil 2 minutes or until slightly thickened. Remove from heat, stir in vanilla, and top with crumble.

4 For peak flavors, let stand for at least two hours to absorb flavors and blend. You can store this dish in the refrigerator for up to 3 days.

Calories 205
Calories from fat 80
Total fat 9.0 g
Saturated fat 0.8 g
Trans fat 0.0 g

Cholesterol 0 mg
Sodium 40 mg
Total carbohydrate 30 g
Dietary fiber 3 g
Sugars 22 g
Protein 2 g

EXCHANGES
PER SERVING
2 carbohydrate
1½ fat

Flavorful tip As with most fruit pies, the flavors improve and mellow if it is allowed to stand overnight or for at least 4 hours. Do not cook the pie crumble any longer than directed because it will become very crunchy while cooling.

FRESH AND DRIED FRUIT GINGER CRUMBLE

YIELD 10 servings | **SERVING SIZE** ½ cup

Mixing sweet, concentrated candied ginger with pineapple and nectarines makes this crumble explode with flavor. Serve it warm or at room temperature.

FILLING

- 4 ripe fresh pineapple slices, ½ inch thick, chopped (about 3 cups total)
- 1 ripe medium nectarine or pear, peeled, pitted/cored, and chopped (about 1 cup total)
- 1 tablespoon packed brown sugar substitute blend
- ⅓ cup golden raisins
- 1 ounce chopped candied ginger (about 3 tablespoons)
- ¼ cup water
- 2 teaspoons cornstarch

  Canola oil cooking spray

TOPPING

- 12 gingersnap cookies
- 2 tablespoons canola oil
- 1 tablespoon packed brown sugar substitute blend
- ¼ teaspoon ground nutmeg

1 Preheat oven to 350°F.

2 Combine filling ingredients in a medium bowl and toss gently, yet thoroughly, until cornstarch is dissolved. Place in an 11 × 7-inch glass baking dish coated with cooking spray; set aside.

3 Place gingersnaps in a small plastic bag and crush cookies using a meat mallet or the bottom of a can until they have a coarse texture. Place in a small mixing bowl and add remaining topping ingredients. Stir to blend thoroughly and sprinkle evenly over fruit.

4 Bake, uncovered, 30 minutes or until fruit is bubbly. Remove from heat and let stand 10 minutes to absorb flavors.

Fast tip To serve only five, divide the recipe in half and bake in a loaf pan as directed. Store cooled leftovers covered in the refrigerator for up to 2 days. Reheat leftovers in the microwave and serve over fat-free ice cream or banana slices.

Calories 125	Cholesterol 0 mg
Calories from fat 35	Sodium 55 mg
Total fat 4.0 g	Total carbohydrate 23 g
Saturated fat 0.4 g	Dietary fiber 1 g
Trans fat 0.0 g	Sugars 15 g
	Protein 1 g

EXCHANGES PER SERVING
1½ carbohydrate
½ fat

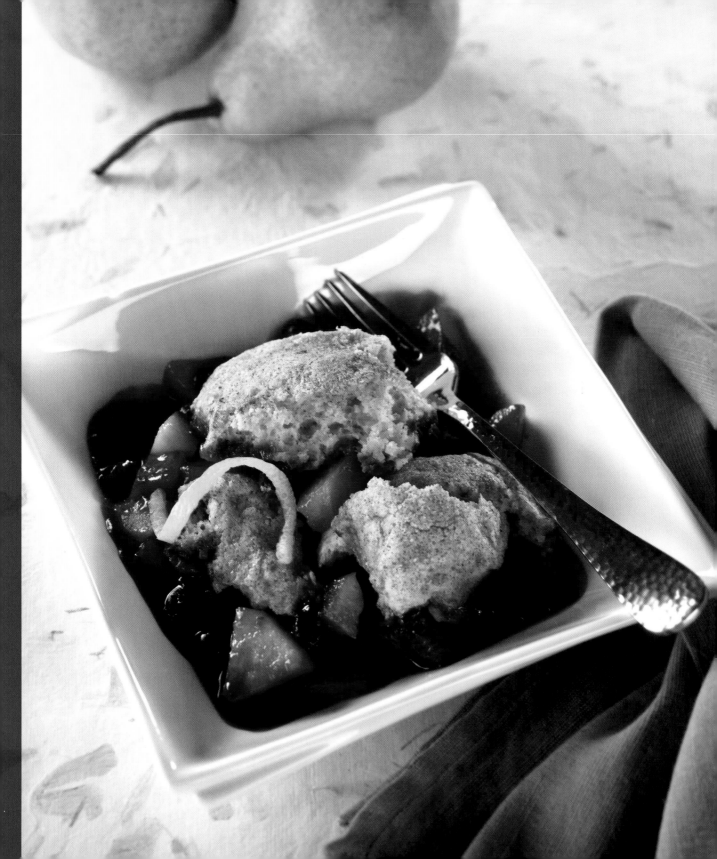

BLUEBERRY-LEMON COUNTRY COBBLER

YIELD 8 servings | **SERVING SIZE** ½ cup

Adding diced pear and a generous amount of fresh lemon zest gives a true freshness to this extraordinary fruit cobbler.

Canola oil cooking spray

FILLING

- 3 tablespoons sugar
- 1 tablespoon cornstarch
- ¼ cup water
- 1 lb fresh (or partially thawed frozen) blueberries
- 1 ripe medium pear, peeled, halved, cored, and diced
- 1 tablespoon lemon zest

TOPPING

- ¾ cup white whole-wheat flour, spooned into measuring cup and leveled
- 2½ tablespoons sugar
- 1 teaspoon baking powder
- ½ cup fat-free buttermilk
- 2 tablespoons canola oil
- 1 egg white
- 1 teaspoon lemon zest
- ¼ teaspoon ground cinnamon

1 Preheat oven to 400°F.

2 Coat an 11 × 7-inch baking pan with cooking spray.

3 Combine sugar, cornstarch, and water in a large nonreactive saucepan. Stir until cornstarch is completely dissolved, then stir in berries and pears. Bring to a boil over medium-high heat and boil 1 full minute. Remove from heat and stir in 1 tablespoon zest. Place fruit mixture in the baking pan.

4 Combine flour, 2 tablespoons sugar, and baking powder in a medium bowl. Combine buttermilk, canola oil, egg white, and remaining 1 teaspoon zest in a small bowl. Add buttermilk mixture to flour mixture and stir until just blended. Spoon batter into eight small mounds on top of the filling. Mix remaining sugar with cinnamon and sprinkle on top of cobbler. Bake 20–25 minutes or until filling is bubbly and a wooden pick inserted into the topping comes out clean. Let stand 20 minutes to absorb flavors.

Fresh tip The canola oil makes the topping spread, creating a rustic cobbler appearance. Blueberries may be substituted with raspberries or mixed berries.

Calories 165	Cholesterol 0 mg
Calories from fat 35	Sodium 70 mg
Total fat 4.0 g	Total carbohydrate 31 g
Saturated fat 0.3 g	Dietary fiber 4 g
Trans fat 0.0 g	Sugars 17 g
	Protein 3 g

EXCHANGES PER SERVING
2 carbohydrate
1 fat

HOMESTYLE SHORTCAKES

YIELD 4 servings | **SERVING SIZE** 1 shortcake + ½ cup fruit mixture

These cute cakes stack up to a sensational, summery dessert. Buttermilk gives them richness, while fruit on top offers contrasting lightness.

TOPPING

2 cups fresh (or thawed frozen) blackberries

1 tablespoon pourable sugar substitute

1 teaspoon canola oil

½ teaspoon vanilla extract

¼–½ cup fat-free whipped topping (optional)

SHORTCAKES

1 cup white whole-wheat flour, spooned into measuring cup and leveled

2 tablespoons pourable sugar substitute

1 teaspoon baking powder

1 teaspoon ground cinnamon

⅓ cup fat-free buttermilk

2 tablespoons canola oil

1 egg white

Canola oil cooking spray

1 Preheat oven to 450°F. Combine topping ingredients, except whipped topping, in a medium bowl and set aside.

2 Combine flour, sugar substitute, baking powder, and cinnamon in another medium bowl. Combine buttermilk, canola oil, and egg white in a small bowl and whisk until well blended. Add to flour mixture and stir until just blended.

3 Coat a nonstick cookie sheet and the back of a spoon with cooking spray. Spoon batter onto cookie sheet in four mounds. Flatten mounds with back of spoon to about 3 inches in diameter. Bake 8 minutes or until a wooden pick comes out clean.

4 Let stand 10 minutes before cutting each in half horizontally. Place bottom of shortcakes on individual dessert plates, spoon equal amounts of topping on each, and place shortcake tops on top. Spoon whipped topping on each, if desired.

Calories 245
Calories from fat 80
Total fat 9.0 g
    Saturated fat 0.7 g
    Trans fat 0.0 g

Cholesterol 0 mg
Sodium 130 mg
Total carbohydrate 34 g
    Dietary fiber 8 g
    Sugars 6 g
Protein 7 g

EXCHANGES PER SERVING
2 carbohydrate
2 fat

Fresh tip The shortcakes will spread slightly during the cooking process. Mixed berries, strawberries, blueberries, or frozen peaches can be substituted for blackberries.

SPICED BERRY SAUCE

Adding canola oil to this versatile topping not only gives it a smooth texture, but also makes it glisten with photogenic quality. Serve the sauce over fat-free ice cream, fruit, or angel food cake...whatever may benefit from berry good flavor.

- 1 lb fresh (or partially thawed frozen) mixed berries
- 1 tablespoon canola oil
- 1½ tablespoons orange zest
- ½ teaspoon ground cinnamon
- 1 teaspoon vanilla extract
- 1 cup water
- ⅓ cup sugar

1 Combine all ingredients, except water and sugar, in a shallow pan, such as a 9-inch, deep-dish glass pie pan and set aside.

2 Bring water to a boil over high heat in a small saucepan. Add sugar and cook until sugar dissolves. Pour hot sugar mixture over fruit mixture and mix gently, yet thoroughly, to blend. Let stand 30 minutes.

3 Sauce can be served on melon slices, banana slices, fat-free ice cream, angel food cake, waffles, or French toast.

Flavorful tip This technique allows the strawberries to soften without disintegrating and the flavors of the orange to be released.

Calories 50
  Calories from fat 15
Total fat 1.5 g
  Saturated fat 0.1 g
  Trans fat 0.0 g

Cholesterol 0 mg
Sodium 0 mg
Total carbohydrate 10 g
  Dietary fiber 2 g
  Sugars 8 g
Protein 0 g

EXCHANGES
PER SERVING
½ carbohydrate

MELON INFUSED WITH MINT AND LIME

YIELD 4 servings | **SERVING SIZE** 1 cup melon

Whether you use watermelon or honeydew, the melon will sponge up the minty lime juice, giving every bite of this healthy dessert a burst of freshness!

2 teaspoons lime zest

¼ cup fresh lime juice

1 tablespoon canola oil

2 teaspoons sugar

⅛ teaspoon peppermint extract (optional)

4 cups watermelon or honeydew melon cubes

¼ cup chopped mint leaves

1 Combine zest, juice, canola oil, sugar, and peppermint extract in a small bowl and whisk until well blended.

2 Place 1 cup melon on each of four dessert plates, cocktail glasses, or wine goblets. Spoon equal amounts of lime mixture over each and top with chopped mint. Serve immediately for peak flavors and texture.

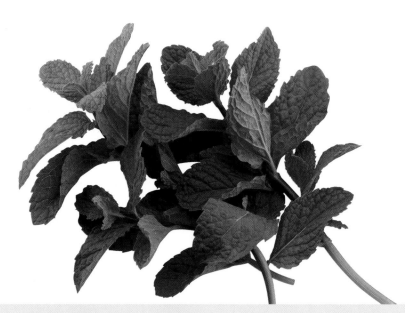

Calories 90	Cholesterol 0 mg	
Calories from fat 35	Sodium 0 mg	
Total fat 4.0 g	Total carbohydrate 15 g	**EXCHANGES PER SERVING**
Saturated fat 0.3 g	Dietary fiber 1 g	1 fruit
Trans fat 0.0 g	Sugars 12 g	1 fat
	Protein 1 g	

Fresh tip Whenever combining fresh herbs with canola oil, use the oil immediately; do not store it in the refrigerator. Oil is anaerobic, meaning it prevents any moisture in the herbs from evaporating, which can cause bacteria to develop.

TRADITIONAL ROLLED SUGAR COOKIES

YIELD 16 servings | **SERVING SIZE** 3 cookies

Try the great technique below with all of your rolled cookie recipes. It's so easy, you'll never go back to your old ways.

¾ cup sugar

½ cup canola oil

1 teaspoon baking powder

¼ teaspoon salt

2 egg whites

1 teaspoon vanilla extract

1⅓ cups all-purpose flour, spooned into measuring cups and leveled

⅔ cup white whole-wheat flour, spooned into measuring cup and leveled

1 Combine the sugar and canola oil in a medium bowl. Using an electric mixer, beat on medium speed until well blended. Beat in remaining ingredients, except flours, scraping sides occasionally. Reduce mixer to low speed and gradually add flours.

2 Place the dough on parchment paper (about 12 × 18 inches), top with another sheet of parchment paper, and roll to ⅛-inch thickness. Place parchment paper with dough on a large cookie sheet and refrigerate 30 minutes.

3 Preheat oven to 375°F.

4 Remove top sheet of parchment paper. Using a 2-inch cookie or biscuit cutter, cut dough into desired shapes, and place them on an ungreased cookie sheet, about ½ inch apart. Sprinkle lightly with sugar and bake 6 minutes or until edges are firm and bottoms are lightly browned. Remove from cookie sheet and place on a wire rack to cool completely. Repeat with remaining cookie dough.

Fast tip Be sure to roll out the dough between the parchment paper and then chill it for easy handling and cutting.

Calories 155
  Calories from fat 65
Total fat 7.0 g
  Saturated fat 0.5 g
  Trans fat 0.0 g

Cholesterol 0 mg
Sodium 65 mg
Total carbohydrate 21 g
  Dietary fiber 1 g
  Sugars 10 g
Protein 2 g

EXCHANGES PER SERVING
1½ carbohydrate
1 fat

TOFFEE-PECAN TOPPED COOKIES

YIELD 16 servings | **SERVING SIZE** 3 cookies

These decadent drop cookies will drop out of sight if they're left on the counter without supervision!

Canola oil cooking spray

⅔ cup white whole-wheat flour, spooned into measuring cup and leveled

2 teaspoons baking powder

½ teaspoon baking soda

¼ teaspoon salt

½ cup packed dark brown sugar

⅓ cup sugar

¼ cup egg substitute

3 tablespoons canola oil

1 teaspoon vanilla, butter, and nut flavoring or 2 teaspoons vanilla extract

TOPPING

¼ cup (1 ounce) pecan pieces, toasted and finely chopped

¼ cup toffee bits

1 Preheat oven to 350°F. Coat a baking sheet with cooking spray.

2 Combine flour, baking powder, baking soda, and salt in a medium bowl; set aside.

3 Combine brown sugar, sugar, egg substitute, canola oil, and vanilla flavoring in another medium bowl. With an electric mixer on high speed, cream together until smooth and fluffy.

4 Reduce to medium-low speed, gradually add flour mixture to creamed mixture, and beat until well blended. Drop mixture 2 inches apart by level teaspoons onto a cookie sheet. Combine nuts and toffee in a small bowl. Top each cookie with ½ teaspoon nut mixture. Bake 7 minutes. Let stand 1 minute on the cookie sheet before removing with a metal spatula. Cool on a wire rack.

Calories 120	Cholesterol 0 mg	
Calories from fat 45	Sodium 150 mg	**EXCHANGES PER SERVING**
Total fat 5.0 g	Total carbohydrate 18 g	
Saturated fat 0.9 g	Dietary fiber 1 g	1 carbohydrate
Trans fat 0.0 g	Sugars 13 g	1 fat
	Protein 1 g	

Flavorful tip The "vanilla, butter, and nut flavoring" is one flavoring, not three separate ones. It is sold next to vanilla extract in most supermarkets and gives the cookies a butterscotch flavor. Don't like toffee? Use mini chocolate chips instead!

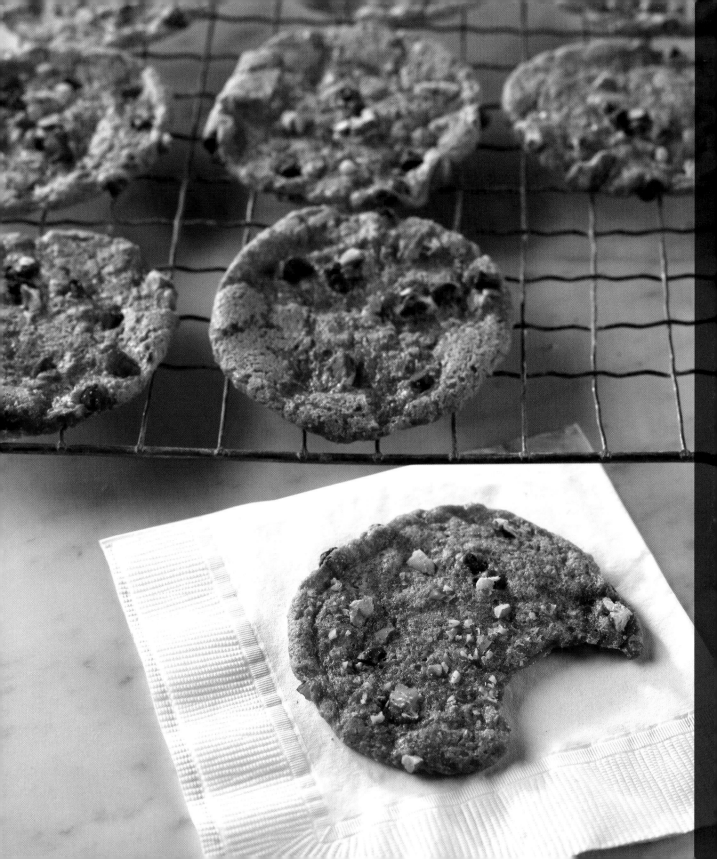

STICKY, CRUNCHY CEREAL ROUNDS

YIELD 12 servings | **SERVING SIZE** 1 round

These cookies are like cereal treats, but are loaded with fiber and other good stuff. Because the recipe is made with canola oil, the rounds will remain chewy and not dry out.

Canola oil cooking spray

¼ cup (1 ounce) chopped pecans or walnuts

1¼ cups mini marshmallows

¼ cup light corn syrup

2 tablespoons canola oil

8 ounces whole-grain granola cereal clusters with dried fruits and nuts

6 dried apricot halves, chopped

1–2 teaspoons orange zest

1 Coat a 12-cup nonstick muffin pan with cooking spray; set aside.

2 Heat a large saucepan over medium heat. Add nuts and cook 3 minutes or until lightly browned and fragrant, stirring constantly. Reduce heat to low; add marshmallows, syrup, and canola oil to pan. Stir until marshmallows are completely melted and add cereal, apricots, and zest. Stir quickly to blend.

3 Remove from heat and spoon equal amounts of cereal mixture into each of 12 muffin tins. Press down lightly with your fingertips or the back of a spoon coated with cooking spray to prevent sticking while leveling out rounds. Let stand 10 minutes. Remove rounds from pan and store in an airtight container.

Calories 160	Cholesterol 0 mg	
Calories from fat 65	Sodium 50 mg	**EXCHANGES PER SERVING**
Total fat 7.0 g	Total carbohydrate 25 g	1½ carbohydrate
Saturated fat 0.6 g	Dietary fiber 3 g	1 fat
Trans fat 0.0 g	Sugars 12 g	
	Protein 3 g	

Fast tip This is a very fast-paced dish to assemble, so be sure to have all of the ingredients ready before beginning.

APRICOT-CRANBERRY NUT SQUARES

YIELD 12 servings | **SERVING SIZE** 2 squares

These colorful cookies look as good as they taste! Chewy, jammy, nutty...
delicious.

1 cup whole-wheat flour, spooned into measuring cup and leveled

½ teaspoon baking powder

¼ teaspoon salt

¼ teaspoon ground cardamom or ¼ teaspoon ground cinnamon

½ cup orange juice

⅓ cup canola oil

¼ cup egg substitute

¼ cup packed brown sugar substitute blend

2 ounces chopped walnuts, pistachios, or slivered almonds

½ cup apricot fruit spread

¼ cup dried cranberries

1 Preheat oven to 350°F.

2 Line an 11 × 7-inch glass baking pan with enough foil to overhang the edges slightly.

3 Combine flour, baking powder, salt, and cardamom or cinnamon in a medium bowl.

4 Combine juice, canola oil, egg substitute, and sugar in another medium bowl and whisk until well blended. Add to flour mixture and stir until just blended. Spoon batter into the baking pan, spread evenly over all, and bake 20–21 minutes or until a wooden pick inserted near the center comes out clean. Place baking pan on a wire cooling rack and cool completely.

5 Remove baked cookie base from foil and place on a cutting board. Heat a medium skillet over medium-high heat. Add nuts and cook 2 minutes or until fragrant, stirring frequently. Remove from skillet; set aside to cool.

6 To skillet, add fruit spread and heat over medium-high heat until slightly melted, stirring constantly. Remove from heat and spread evenly over cookie base. Top with nuts and cranberries. Cool before cutting into 24 squares. Refrigerate leftovers.

Fresh tip To make these bars even prettier, cut each square in half diagonally.

Calories 175
    Calories from fat 80
Total fat 9.0 g
    Saturated fat 0.8 g
    Trans fat 0.0 g

Cholesterol 0 mg
Sodium 80 mg
Total carbohydrate 22 g
    Dietary fiber 2 g
    Sugars 12 g
Protein 3 g

EXCHANGES PER SERVING
1½ carbohydrate
2 fat

RICH, WARM BROWNIE WEDGES
with Java Cream

YIELD 8 servings | **SERVING SIZE** 1/8 brownie + 1/4 cup berries

Dense wedges of chewy chocolate are paired with a sweet coffee-flavored cream and fresh berries.

WEDGES

Canola oil cooking spray

2/3 cup all-purpose flour, spooned into measuring cup and leveled

1/3 cup white whole-wheat flour, spooned into measuring cup and leveled

1/2 cup cocoa powder

1 1/2 teaspoons baking powder

1 tablespoon instant coffee granules

1/8 teaspoon salt

1/2 cup packed brown sugar substitute blend

1/3 cup canola oil

1/2 cup egg substitute

2 teaspoons vanilla extract

CREAM

2 tablespoons water

1 teaspoon instant coffee granules

4 ounces fat-free whipped topping

1 cup fresh raspberries

1 cup blackberries or blueberries

1 Preheat oven to 325°F. Coat a 9-inch, nonstick spring-form pan or cake pan with cooking spray.

2 Combine flours, cocoa and baking powders, 1 tablespoon coffee granules, and salt in a medium bowl.

3 Combine sugar, canola oil, egg substitute, and vanilla in another medium bowl; mix well. Add sugar mixture to flour mixture and stir until just blended. Batter will be very thick. Spoon into the bottom of the pan; spread evenly by coating the back of a spoon with cooking spray. Bake for 11 minutes or until slightly puffed. (Mixture will not be completely cooked at this point, but it will continue to cook while standing without overcooking and drying out.) Place the pan on a wire rack and let cool for 5 minutes. Remove the sides of the pan and gently remove from bottom or leave on bottom and place on a serving plate. Serve warm or at room temperature. When cooled completely, store in an airtight container at room temperature.

4 To make cream, combine water with 1 teaspoon instant coffee granules in a medium bowl and stir until dissolved. Add whipped topping; whisk until a sauce consistency is reached. For thinner sauce, add 1–2 tablespoons water or milk. Refrigerate until needed. To serve, cut into wedges, spoon mocha cream on top, and sprinkle with berries.

Calories 260
  Calories from fat 90
Total fat 10.0 g
  Saturated fat 1.0 g
  Trans fat 0.0 g

Cholesterol 0 mg
Sodium 145 mg
Total carbohydrate 36 g
  Dietary fiber 4 g
  Sugars 16 g
Protein 5 g

EXCHANGES PER SERVING
2 1/2 carbohydrate
2 fat

Fresh tip The secret to a moist brownie is canola oil. It will keep this brownie soft for two days.

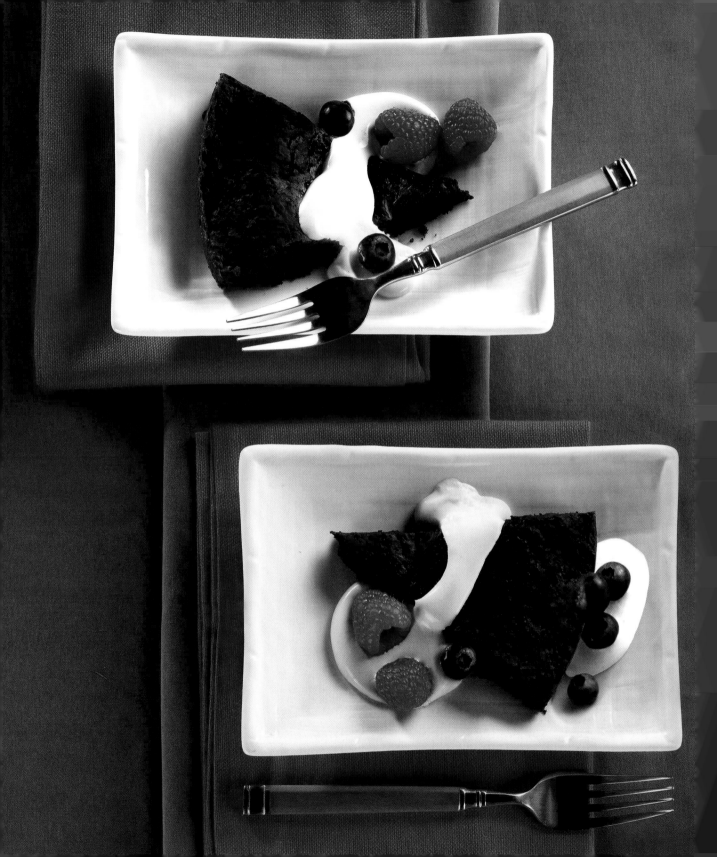

CHOCOLATE FONDUE

YIELD 8 servings | **SERVING SIZE** 2 tablespoons

Fondues are always popular, especially when there's chocolate involved. You'd never know this dish is healthier than traditional chocolate fondue because it's just that good!

- ¼ cup cocoa powder
- 1 cup fat-free evaporated milk
- 1 tablespoon canola oil
- 1½ ounces bittersweet chocolate, chopped
- ¼ cup packed brown sugar substitute blend
- ½ teaspoon vanilla extract (optional)
- 8 wooden picks

1 Whisk together cocoa, milk, and canola oil in a medium saucepan. Place over medium-high heat and bring just to a boil, about 3 minutes. Reduce heat; simmer for 4 minutes or until slightly thickened, stirring frequently. Add chocolate, reduce to low heat, and stir until melted. Remove from heat; whisk in sugar and vanilla.

2 To serve, provide wooden picks for dipping strawberries, bananas, or cubes of angel food cake. Fondue may also be served with biscotti, such as the Almond-Cherry Biscotti, or over fat-free frozen yogurt.

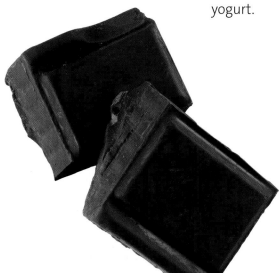

Calories 105
Calories from fat 40
Total fat 4.5 g
Saturated fat 1.5 g
Trans fat 0.0 g

Cholesterol 0 mg
Sodium 40 mg
Total carbohydrate 14 g
Dietary fiber 1 g
Sugars 12 g
Protein 3 g

EXCHANGES PER SERVING
1 carbohydrate
1 fat

Flavorful tip Canola oil adds fluidity to this chocolate fondue so that dipping fruit or cake is easy.

INDEX

A

Almond Cherry Biscotti with Citrus, 36

Apricot-Cranberry Nut Squares, 211

Apricot Hoisin-Glazed Meatballs, 85

Artichoke Frittata with Fresh Vegetable Sauté, 19

Asian Vegetable Slaw, 95

Asparagus-Wheat Berry Salad with Blue Cheese, 106

Asparagus with Creamy Dijon Sauce, 112

B

Baby Spinach and Prosciutto with Sherry Vinaigrette, 97

Baked Acorn Squash with Cranberry-Orange Sauce, 126

Baked Chicken Legs with Creamy Honey-Mustard Dip, 148

Banana Bread with Honey Drizzle, 33

Barley-Artichoke Salad on Romaine, 103

Barley, White Bean, and Artichoke Toss, 181

Basil Focaccia Wedges, 79

Beef Tenderloin and Portobellos with Marsala Sauce, 175

Black Bean Burgers with Avocado-Lime Mayonnaise, 183

Black Bean, Jalapeño, and Yellow Rice Salad, 52

Black Bean Skillet with Butternut Squash, 184

Black Bean Tortilla Rounds, 29

Black Beans with Green Chile Sauce, 113

Black-Eyed Peas with Jalapeño and Tomatoes, 114

Blueberry-Lemon Country Cobbler, 203

Bulgur and Rosemary-Edamame Salad, 51

Buttermilk Pancakes with Fresh Strawberry-Orange Topping, 27

C

Cajun Pile-Ups with Pepper Sauce, 58

Canola Granola, 41

Central American-Style Beef, 173

Chicken and Artichokes with Pasta, 155

Chicken with Roasted Red Pepper Sauce, 152

Chocolate Fondue, 214
Chocolate Mint Pie with Espresso Sauce, 199
Classic Tuna Casserole, 142
Coffee-Crusted Sirloin Steak, 172
Corn and Skillet-Roasted Poblano Soup, 44
Creamy Apricot-Mango Smoothies, 39
Creamy Beef, Mushrooms, and Noodles, 178
Creamy Black Bean Stack Dip, 73
Creamy Pumpkin-Apple Bisque, 48
Crispy Baked Zucchini Spears with Lemon, 76
Crispy Crunchy Oven-Fried Okra, 124
Crunchy Chicken-Cilantro Lettuce Wraps, 55
Crunchy Red Pepper-Ginger Relish with
    Cucumber Rounds, 71
Cumin'd Lentils and Carrots, 121
Curried Sweet Potato and Peanut Stew, 188

D
Deviled Crab Cakes with Spicy Sauce, 138
Drunken Beef Goulash, 177

E
English Muffin Pile-Ups, 22

F
Fish Tacos with Avocado Salsa, 146
French Toast with Blueberries and Creamy
    Apricot Sauce, 24
French Toast with Dark Cherry-Pomegranate
    Sauce, 26
Fresh and Dried Fruit Ginger Crumble, 201
Fresh Broccoli and Dried Cranberry Salad, 94
Fresh Herb and Spinach Quiche, 18
Fresh Spinach and Sweet Tomato Omelet with
    Feta, 20

G
Garlic Snow Peas with Cilantro, 123
Garlic White Bean Soup with Smoked
    Sausage, 47
Glazed Pineapple-Orange Bundt Cake, 194
Greek Garbanzo Salsa Salad, 91
Greek Pepperoncini Pitas, 57
Green Beans with Spicy Mustard Sauce, 119
Grill Pan Chicken with Fiery Mango-Ginger
    Salsa, 151

Grilled Cinnamon-Pear Sandwiches, 28
Grilled Flank Steak with Balsamic Vinegar and
    Red Wine, 171
Grilled Shrimp with Sweet Hot Sauce, 140
Grilled Tuna Niçoise Salad, 53

H
Ham and Lentil Soup with Cloves, 45
Harvest Pumpkin Pie, 198
Hash Browns with Ham and Chunky
    Vegetables, 31
Hearty Minestrone with Sausage, 46
High-Roasted Onions, 135
Hoisin Orange Pork on Asian Vegetables, 166
Homestyle Shortcakes, 204
Hometown Turkey Meatloaf, 159

I
Italian-Style Sub with Dijon-Garlic Spread, 60

J
Jambalaya with Smoked Turkey Sausage and
    Chicken, 156
Jicama and Sweet Lemon Salad, 93

L
Layered Mexican Casserole, 180
Lentil Tortillas, 65
Lime-Infused Halibut with Ginger Relish, 143
Lime-Zested Tomatillo-Black Bean Salad, 89

M
Mango-Banana Phyllo Nests, 196
Marinated Italian Vegetable Toss, 68
Melon Infused with Mint and Lime, 206
Mini Corn Cakes with Chipotle Aioli, 77
Mini Fruit Tarts with Cheesecake Filling, 195
Mini Greek Chicken Kabobs, 84
Mini Potatoes with Caramelized Onions and
    Blue Cheese, 74
Mini Vegetable Panini, 80
Mixed Greens, String Beans, and Walnuts with
    White Wine-Raspberry Vinaigrette, 100

O
Oatmeal Breakfast Cookies, 35
Open-Faced Sloppy Joes, 64

P

Panko-Parmesan Chicken with Capers, 153

Poached Egg-English Muffin Stacks with Creamy Lemon Sauce, 23

Pork Medallions with Rich Onion Sauce, 165

Pork Sliders with Raspberry Mustard Sauce, 82

Pork Tenderloin, Potatoes, and Horseradish-Mustard Seed Sauce, 163

Pork Tenderloin with Sweet Soy Marinade, 164

Provençal Chicken with White Wine, Garlic, and Apricots, 149

Q

Quinoa and Browned Onion Salad with Apples, 105

R

Red Wine-Braised Beef with Vegetables, 176

Rich, Warm Brownie Wedges with Java Cream, 212

Roasted Beet and Carrot Salad, 98

Roasted Root Vegetables with Balsamic Reduction, 132

Roasted Salmon with Adobo Cream Sauce, 144

Roasted Turkey with Rosemary and Sage, 158

Rosemary Pork Chops with Tomato-Caper Topping, 170

S

Sausage and Country Vegetables on Grits, 32

Sausage and Veggie Breakfast Casserole, 21

Sautéed Apple-Raisin Oatmeal, 38

Scallops with Parmesan Pasta, 139

Sesame Thai Toss with Peanut Lime Sauce, 191

Shredded Cajun Pork and Grits, 168

Simple Fresh Herb Salad, 101

Skillet Broccoli with Tangy Sweet Sauce, 116

Skillet Pie with Oat-Pecan Crumble, 200

Skillet Turkey Ham with Curried Apples and Onions, 160

Slow Cooker Smoky Pork Buns, 169

Soy-Marinated Mushrooms with Cilantro and Basil, 75

Spiced Berry Sauce, 205

Spicy Corn with Poblano Peppers, 117

Spicy Mediterranean White Bean Hummus, 70

Spinach and Mushroom Barley Pilaf, 130

Spinach Salad with Grilled and Fresh Fruit, 109

Spring Greens with Chicken and Sweet Pomegranate Vinaigrette, 56

Stewed Eggplant, Tomatoes, and Fresh Basil, 118

Sticky, Crunchy Cereal Rounds, 210

Stuffed Portobello Caps with Parmesan Crumb Topping, 125

Sweet and Crispy Cucumber-Anaheim Salad, 102

Sweet Grape Tomato and Poblano Salad, 90

Sweet Home Chili on Spaghetti Squash, 185

Sweet Pineapple-Ginger Slaw, 96

Sweet Potatoes with Caramelized Sherry Onions, 133

Sweet Spice-Rubbed Chicken, 154

Sweet Tomato Creole Tilapia, 145

T

Thyme-Roasted Pork Loin with Peach-Raspberry Sauce, 161

Toasted Pecan Quinoa with Red Peppers, 190

Toasted Sesame Seed Quinoa, 128

Toffee-Pecan Topped Cookies, 208

Traditional Rolled Sugar Cookies, 207

Tuna Kabobs with Mild Wasabi Cream, 141

Turkey-Swiss Panini, 61

Turnip Greens with Smoked Sausage, 120

V

Vegetable Pasta with Tapenade and Pine Nuts, 186

Vegetable Penne Salad with Feta, 50

Vegetarian Sandwich with Sun-Dried Tomato Spread, 62

W

West Indies Shrimp and Jalapeño Rounds, 81

White Bean and Roasted Red Pepper Salad, 88

Whole-Grain Blueberry Muffins, 34

Wilted Kale Salad, 107

Y

Yellow Rice and Red Pepper Tosser, 129

Z

Zucchini Boats, 134

RECIPES BY DISH TYPE OR MAIN INGREDIENT

ARTICHOKES

Artichoke Frittata with Fresh Vegetable Sauté, 19

Barley-Artichoke Salad on Romaine, 103

Barley, White Bean, and Artichoke Toss, 181

Chicken and Artichokes with Pasta, 155

Greek Garbanzo Salsa Salad, 91

Marinated Italian Vegetable Toss, 68

Vegetable Penne Salad with Feta, 50

BARLEY

Barley-Artichoke Salad on Romaine, 103

Barley, White Bean, and Artichoke Toss, 181

Spinach and Mushroom Barley Pilaf, 130

BEANS (PULSES)

Barley, White Bean, and Artichoke Toss, 181

Black Bean Burgers with Avocado-Lime Mayonnaise, 183

Black Bean, Jalapeño, and Yellow Rice Salad, 52

Black Bean Skillet with Butternut Squash, 184

Black Bean Tortilla Rounds, 29

Black Beans with Green Chile Sauce, 113

Black-Eyed Peas with Jalapeño and Tomatoes, 114

Creamy Black Bean Stack Dip, 73

Curried Sweet Potato and Peanut Stew, 188

Garlic White Bean Soup with Smoked Sausage, 47

Greek Garbanzo Salsa Salad, 91

Ham and Lentil Soup with Cloves, 45

Lentil Tortillas, 65

Lime-Zested Tomatillo-Black Bean Salad, 89

Marinated Italian Vegetable Toss, 68

Sweet Home Chili on Spaghetti Squash, 185

White Bean and Roasted Red Pepper Salad, 88

BEEF

Apricot Hoisin-Glazed Meatballs, 85

Beef Tenderloin and Portobellos with Marsala Sauce, 175

Central American-Style Beef, 173

Coffee-Crusted Sirloin Steak, 172

Creamy Beef, Mushrooms, and Noodles, 178

Drunken Beef Goulash, 177

Grilled Flank Steak with Balsamic Vinegar and Red Wine, 171

Layered Mexican Casserole, 180

Red Wine-Braised Beef with Vegetables, 176

BREADS AND MUFFINS

Banana Bread with Honey Drizzle, 33

Basil Focaccia Wedges, 79

Whole-Grain Blueberry Muffins, 34

CAKES

Glazed Pineapple-Orange Bundt Cake, 194

Homestyle Shortcakes, 204

Mini Fruit Tarts with Cheesecake Filling, 195

CASSEROLES

Classic Tuna Casserole, 142

Layered Mexican Casserole, 180

Sausage and Veggie Breakfast Casserole, 21

CEREALS (OATMEAL, GRANOLA, AND GRITS)

Canola Granola, 41

Sausage and Country Vegetables on Grits, 32

Sautéed Apple-Raisin Oatmeal, 38

Shredded Cajun Pork and Grits, 168

Sticky, Crunchy Cereal Rounds, 210

CHICKEN

Baked Chicken Legs with Creamy Honey-Mustard Dip, 148

Bulgur and Rosemary-Edamame Salad, 51

Chicken and Artichokes with Pasta, 155

Chicken with Roasted Red Pepper Sauce, 152

Crunchy Chicken-Cilantro Lettuce Wraps, 55

Grill Pan Chicken with Fiery Mango-Ginger Salsa, 151

Jambalaya with Smoked Turkey Sausage and Chicken, 156

Mini Greek Chicken Kabobs, 84

Panko-Parmesan Chicken with Capers, 153

Provençal Chicken with White Wine, Garlic, and Apricots, 149

Spring Greens with Chicken and Sweet Pomegranate Vinaigrette, 56

Sweet Spice-Rubbed Chicken, 154

CHILES

Black Bean, Jalapeño, and Yellow Rice Salad, 52

Black-Eyed Peas with Jalapeño and Tomatoes, 114

Cajun Pile-Ups with Pepper Sauce, 58

Corn and Skillet-Roasted Poblano Soup, 44

Greek Pepperoncini Pitas, 57

Lime-Zested Tomatillo-Black Bean Salad, 89

Spicy Corn with Poblano Peppers, 117

Sweet and Crispy Cucumber-Anaheim Salad, 102

Sweet Grape Tomato and Poblano Salad, 90

West Indies Shrimp and Jalapeño Rounds, 81

CHOCOLATE

Chocolate Fondue, 214

Chocolate Mint Pie with Espresso Sauce, 199

Rich, Warm Brownie Wedges with Java Cream, 212

COOKIES

Almond Cherry Biscotti with Citrus, 36

Apricot-Cranberry Nut Squares, 211

Oatmeal Breakfast Cookies, 35

Sticky, Crunchy Cereal Rounds, 210

Toffee-Pecan Topped Cookies, 208

Traditional Rolled Sugar Cookies, 207

DIPS

Chocolate Fondue, 214

Creamy Black Bean Stack Dip, 73

Crunchy Red Pepper-Ginger Relish with Cucumber Rounds, 71

Spiced Berry Sauce, 205

Spicy Mediterranean White Bean Hummus, 70

EGGS

Artichoke Frittata with Fresh Vegetable Sauté, 19

English Muffin Pile-Ups, 22

Fresh Herb and Spinach Quiche, 18

Fresh Spinach and Sweet Tomato Omelet with Feta, 20

Poached Egg-English Muffin Stacks with Creamy Lemon Sauce, 23

FISH

Classic Tuna Casserole, 142

Fish Tacos with Avocado Salsa, 146

Grilled Tuna Niçoise Salad, 53

Lime-Infused Halibut with Ginger Relish, 143

Roasted Salmon with Adobo Cream Sauce, 144

Sweet Tomato Creole Tilapia, 145

Tuna Kabobs with Mild Wasabi Cream, 141

FRUIT

Buttermilk Pancakes with Fresh Strawberry-Orange Topping, 27

Creamy Apricot-Mango Smoothies, 39

French Toast with Blueberries and Creamy Apricot Sauce, 24

French Toast with Dark Cherry-Pomegranate Sauce, 26

Melon Infused with Mint and Lime, 206

Sautéed Apple-Raisin Oatmeal, 38

Skillet Turkey Ham with Curried Apples and Onions, 160

Spinach Salad with Grilled and Fresh Fruit, 109

MUSHROOMS

Beef Tenderloin and Portobellos with Marsala Sauce, 175

Creamy Beef, Mushrooms, and Noodles, 178

Soy-Marinated Mushrooms with Cilantro and Basil, 75

Spinach and Mushroom Barley Pilaf, 130

Stuffed Portobello Caps with Parmesan Crumb Topping, 125

NUTS

Almond Cherry Biscotti with Citrus, 36

Apricot-Cranberry Nut Squares, 211

Curried Sweet Potato and Peanut Stew, 188

Mixed Greens, String Beans, and Walnuts with White Wine-Raspberry Vinaigrette, 100

Sesame Thai Toss with Peanut Lime Sauce, 191

Toasted Pecan Quinoa with Red Peppers, 190

Toffee-Pecan Topped Cookies, 208

Vegetable Pasta with Tapenade and Pine Nuts, 186

ONIONS

High-Roasted Onions, 135

Mini Potatoes with Caramelized Onions and Blue Cheese, 74

Pork Medallions with Rich Onion Sauce, 165

Quinoa and Browned Onion Salad with Apples, 105

Skillet Turkey Ham with Curried Apples and Onions, 160

Sweet Potatoes with Caramelized Sherry Onions, 133

PANCAKES/FRENCH TOAST

Buttermilk Pancakes with Fresh Strawberry-Orange Topping, 27

French Toast with Blueberries and Creamy Apricot Sauce, 24

French Toast with Dark Cherry-Pomegranate Sauce, 26

PASTA

Chicken and Artichokes with Pasta, 155

Creamy Beef, Mushrooms, and Noodles, 178

Scallops with Parmesan Pasta, 139

Sesame Thai Toss with Peanut Lime Sauce, 191

Vegetable Pasta with Tapenade and Pine Nuts, 186

Vegetable Penne Salad with Feta, 50

PEPPERS

Crunchy Red Pepper-Ginger Relish with Cucumber Rounds, 71

Toasted Pecan Quinoa with Red Peppers, 190

White Bean and Roasted Red Pepper Salad, 88

Yellow Rice and Red Pepper Tosser, 129

PIES/COBBLERS

Blueberry-Lemon Country Cobbler, 203

Chocolate Mint Pie with Espresso Sauce, 199

Fresh and Dried Fruit Ginger Crumble, 201

Harvest Pumpkin Pie, 198

Mango-Banana Phyllo Nests, 196

Skillet Pie with Oat-Pecan Crumble, 200

PORK

Cajun Pile-Ups with Pepper Sauce, 58

Ham and Lentil Soup with Cloves, 45

Hash Browns with Ham and Chunky Vegetables, 31

Hoisin Orange Pork on Asian Vegetables, 166

Poached Egg-English Muffin Stacks with Creamy Lemon Sauce, 23

Pork Medallions with Rich Onion Sauce, 165

Pork Sliders with Raspberry Mustard Sauce, 82

Pork Tenderloin, Potatoes, and Horseradish-Mustard Seed Sauce, 163

Pork Tenderloin with Sweet Soy Marinade, 164

Rosemary Pork Chops with Tomato-Caper Topping, 170

Shredded Cajun Pork and Grits, 168

Slow Cooker Smoky Pork Buns, 169

Thyme-Roasted Pork Loin with Peach-Raspberry Sauce, 161

POTATOES

Curried Sweet Potato and Peanut Stew, 188

Hash Browns with Ham and Chunky Vegetables, 31

Mini Potatoes with Caramelized Onions and Blue Cheese, 74

Pork Tenderloin, Potatoes, and Horseradish-Mustard Seed Sauce, 163

Sweet Potatoes with Caramelized Sherry Onions, 133

QUINOA

Quinoa and Browned Onion Salad with Apples, 105

Toasted Pecan Quinoa with Red Peppers, 190

Toasted Sesame Seed Quinoa, 128

RICE

Black Bean, Jalapeño, and Yellow Rice Salad, 52

Black Bean Skillet with Butternut Squash, 184

Jambalaya with Smoked Turkey Sausage and Chicken, 156

Layered Mexican Casserole, 180

Yellow Rice and Red Pepper Tosser, 129

SALADS

Asian Vegetable Slaw, 95

Asparagus-Wheat Berry Salad with Blue Cheese, 106

Baby Spinach and Prosciutto with Sherry Vinaigrette, 97

Barley-Artichoke Salad on Romaine, 103

Black Bean, Jalapeño, and Yellow Rice Salad, 52

Bulgur and Rosemary-Edamame Salad, 51

Fresh Broccoli and Dried Cranberry Salad, 94

Greek Garbanzo Salsa Salad, 91

Grilled Tuna Niçoise Salad, 53

Jicama and Sweet Lemon Salad, 93

Lime-Zested Tomatillo-Black Bean Salad, 89

Mixed Greens, String Beans, and Walnuts with White Wine-Raspberry Vinaigrette, 100

Quinoa and Browned Onion Salad with Apples, 105

Roasted Beet and Carrot Salad, 98

Simple Fresh Herb Salad, 101

Spinach Salad with Grilled and Fresh Fruit, 109

Spring Greens with Chicken and Sweet Pomegranate Vinaigrette, 56

Sweet and Crispy Cucumber-Anaheim Salad, 102

Sweet Grape Tomato and Poblano Salad, 90

Sweet Pineapple-Ginger Slaw, 96

Vegetable Penne Salad with Feta, 50

White Bean and Roasted Red Pepper Salad, 88

Wilted Kale Salad, 107

SANDWICHES

Black Bean Burgers with Avocado-Lime Mayonnaise, 183

Cajun Pile-Ups with Pepper Sauce, 58

Greek Pepperoncini Pitas, 57

Grilled Cinnamon-Pear Sandwiches, 28

Italian-Style Sub with Dijon-Garlic Spread, 60

Mini Vegetable Panini, 80

Pork Sliders with Raspberry Mustard Sauce, 82

Slow Cooker Smoky Pork Buns, 169

Turkey-Swiss Panini, 61

Vegetarian Sandwich with Sun-Dried Tomato Spread, 62

SAUSAGE

Garlic White Bean Soup with Smoked Sausage, 47

Hearty Minestrone with Sausage, 46

Jambalaya with Smoked Turkey Sausage and Chicken, 156

Sausage and Country Vegetables on Grits, 32

Sausage and Veggie Breakfast Casserole, 21

Turnip Greens with Smoked Sausage, 120

Wilted Kale Salad, 107

SHELLFISH

Deviled Crab Cakes with Spicy Sauce, 138

Grilled Shrimp with Sweet Hot Sauce, 140

Scallops with Parmesan Pasta, 139

West Indies Shrimp and Jalapeño Rounds, 81

SOUPS

Corn and Skillet-Roasted Poblano Soup, 44

Creamy Pumpkin-Apple Bisque, 48

Curried Sweet Potato and Peanut Stew, 188

Garlic White Bean Soup with Smoked Sausage, 47

Ham and Lentil Soup with Cloves, 45

Hearty Minestrone with Sausage, 46

SPINACH

Baby Spinach and Prosciutto with Sherry Vinaigrette, 97

Fresh Herb and Spinach Quiche, 18

Fresh Spinach and Sweet Tomato Omelet with Feta, 20

Spinach and Mushroom Barley Pilaf, 130

Spinach Salad with Grilled and Fresh Fruit, 109

SQUASH

Baked Acorn Squash with Cranberry-Orange Sauce, 126

Black Bean Skillet with Butternut Squash, 184

Creamy Pumpkin-Apple Bisque, 48

Crispy Baked Zucchini Spears with Lemon, 76

Harvest Pumpkin Pie, 198

Sweet Home Chili on Spaghetti Squash, 185

Zucchini Boats, 134

TOMATOES

Artichoke Frittata with Fresh Vegetable Sauté, 19

Black-Eyed Peas with Jalapeño and Tomatoes, 114

Fresh Spinach and Sweet Tomato Omelet with Feta, 20

Rosemary Pork Chops with Tomato-Caper Topping, 170

Stewed Eggplant, Tomatoes, and Fresh Basil, 118

Sweet Grape Tomato and Poblano Salad, 90

Sweet Tomato Creole Tilapia, 145

Vegetarian Sandwich with Sun-Dried Tomato Spread, 62

TURKEY

Garlic White Bean Soup with Smoked Sausage, 47

Greek Pepperoncini Pitas, 57

Hometown Turkey Meatloaf, 159

Jambalaya with Smoked Turkey Sausage and Chicken, 156

Open-Faced Sloppy Joes, 64

Roasted Turkey with Rosemary and Sage, 158

Sausage and Country Vegetables on Grits, 32

Sausage and Veggie Breakfast Casserole, 21

Skillet Turkey Ham with Curried Apples and Onions, 160

Turkey-Swiss Panini, 61

VEGETABLES, GREEN

Asparagus with Creamy Dijon Sauce, 112

Crispy Crunchy Oven-Fried Okra, 124

Crunchy Red Pepper-Ginger Relish with Cucumber Rounds, 71

Garlic Snow Peas with Cilantro, 123

Green Beans with Spicy Mustard Sauce, 119

Hoisin Orange Pork on Asian Vegetables, 166

Marinated Italian Vegetable Toss, 68

Skillet Broccoli with Tangy Sweet Sauce, 116

VEGETABLES, ROOT

Cumin'd Lentils and Carrots, 121

Jicama and Sweet Lemon Salad, 93

Provençal Chicken with White Wine, Garlic, and Apricots, 149

Roasted Beet and Carrot Salad, 98

Roasted Root Vegetables with Balsamic Reduction, 132

Red Wine-Braised Beef with Vegetables, 176

VEGETARIAN MAIN COURSES

Barley, White Bean, and Artichoke Toss, 181

Black Bean Burgers with Avocado-Lime Mayonnaise, 183

Black Bean Skillet with Butternut Squash, 184

Curried Sweet Potato and Peanut Stew, 188

Lentil Tortillas, 65

Sesame Thai Toss with Peanut Lime Sauce, 191

Sweet Home Chili on Spaghetti Squash, 185

Toasted Pecan Quinoa with Red Peppers, 190

Vegetable Pasta with Tapenade and Pine Nuts, 186

Vegetarian Sandwich with Sun-Dried Tomato Spread, 62